Multimodal Interaction Technologies for Training Affective Social Skills

Satoshi Nakamura
Editor

Multimodal Interaction Technologies for Training Affective Social Skills

Springer

Editor
Satoshi Nakamura
Nara Institute of Science and Technology
Ikoma, Nara, Japan

ISBN 978-981-96-1312-0 ISBN 978-981-96-1313-7 (eBook)
https://doi.org/10.1007/978-981-96-1313-7

This Springer imprint is published by the registered company Springer Nature Singapore Pte Ltd.
The registered company address is: 152 Beach Road, #21-01/04 Gateway East, Singapore 189721, Singapore

Preface

Social skills refer to the ability to manage verbal and non-verbal behaviors in interactions with one or more individuals. People who struggle with social interactions often find it difficult to appropriately grasp their social behaviors and understand how others perceive them. Social Skills Training (SST) is a training method developed to improve social interactions and reduce social stress. SST is conducted by clinical psychologists or psychiatrists to ultimately place participants in real social situations, including role-play training that simulates real-world scenarios. This book introduces our research project to develop methods and tools to implement SST using virtual agents as substitutes for human experts and to provide these methods in practice. In our project, we analyze human social skills, break them down into multiple steps, and develop training methods tailored to each step. The targets range from individuals with autism or schizophrenia seeking to improve their social skills to those aiming to enhance their social skills in everyday situations, such as public speaking in schools or workplaces. We are developing a platform with virtual agents that allow participants to role-play social interactions. The project targets both individuals with various social pathologies, such as schizophrenia and autism spectrum disorder (ASD), as well as healthy individuals. In addition to traditional SST, we also explore cognitive-behavioral therapy (CBT), which is used in psychiatry to improve cognitive abilities and alleviate symptoms such as anxiety and depression caused by a lack of social skills and integrate this into the platform.

This research project was a Japan-France international joint ANR-CREST research project. On the Japanese side, it involves Nara Institute of Science and Technology, Osaka University, and Nara Medical University. On the French side, it involves CNRS-ISIR (Institut des Systèmes Intelligents et de Robotique) and CNRS-LISN (Laboratoire Interdisciplinaire des Sciences du Numérique). The SST training system results from joint research between Nara Institute of Science and Technology and Nara Medical University, while the CBT component is based on joint research between Nara Institute of Science and Technology and Osaka University. The virtual agent platform uses a system previously developed by CNRS-ISIR. This book highlights the research outcomes of this project.

The book is composed of six parts. Part one introduces the Social Interaction Theory used in this book, Part two Introduces the Measurement of Social Skills, Part three introduces the Virtual Agent, Part four introduces Interaction and Pedagogical Feedback, and Part five introduces Evaluation.

This research has been conducted with support from the Japan Science and Technology Agency (JST) CREST program on the Japanese side and the Agence Nationale de la Recherche (ANR) on the French side, starting in October 2019 and lasting approximately five years. We sincerely appreciate this project's members and everyone else involved. The project is one of the CREST programs in the area called "Creation and Development of core technologies interfacing human and information environments," which was supervised by Prof. Kenji Mase. We express our gratitude to Prof. Mase and advisors to this project. We also thank the editorial office of Springer for the opportunity and support to publish this book.

Ikoma, Japan Satoshi Nakamura

Contents

Introduces the Social Interaction Theory

Introduction

Satoshi Nakamura

Social skills refer to the ability to manage verbal and non-verbal behaviors in interactions with one or more individuals. People who struggle with social interactions often find it difficult to appropriately grasp their own social behaviors and understand how others perceive them. Social Skills Training (SST) is a training method developed to improve social interactions and reduce social stress. SST is conducted by clinical psychologists or psychiatrists to ultimately place participants in real social situations, including role-play training that simulates real-world scenarios.

Social skills refer to the ability to manage verbal and non-verbal behaviors in interactions with one or more individuals. People who struggle with social interactions often find it difficult to appropriately grasp their own social behaviors and understand how others perceive them. Social Skills Training (SST) is a training method developed to improve social interactions and reduce social stress. SST is conducted by clinical psychologists or psychiatrists to ultimately place participants in real social situations, including role-play training that simulates real-world scenarios.

Our research project aims to develop methods and tools to implement SST using virtual agents as substitutes for human experts and to provide these methods in practice. In our project, we analyze human social skills, break them down into multiple steps, and develop training methods tailored to each step. The target audience ranges from individuals with autism or schizophrenia seeking to improve their social skills, to those aiming to enhance their social skills in everyday situations, such as public speaking in schools or workplaces. We are developing a platform equipped with virtual agents that allows participants to role-play social interactions. The project targets both individuals with various social pathologies, such as schizophrenia and autism spectrum disorder (ASD), as well as healthy individuals. In addition to traditional SST, we also explore cognitive-behavioral therapy (CBT), which is used in

S. Nakamura (✉)
Nara Institute of Science and Technology, Nara, Japan
e-mail: s-nakamura@is.naist.jp

S. Nakamura (ed.), *Multimodal Interaction Technologies for Training Affective Social Skills*, https://doi.org/10.1007/978-981-96-1313-7_1

psychiatry to improve cognitive abilities and alleviate symptoms such as anxiety and depression caused by a lack of social skills, and integrate this into the platform.

Virtual agents simulating one-on-one SST as a tool for helping human participants acquire social skills (e.g., to gain confidence in job interviews) have been researched before. However, these studies often focus on limited interactions, such as virtual interviewers for job interview practice, or use virtual agents with limited interactive functions, targeting a narrow range of users.

In this study, we design conversational virtual agents to take on various roles and scenarios. Depending on the scenario, they function as colleagues, co-presenters, or members of an audience. These agents are designed to be autonomous entities capable of interacting with human users. They are implemented to exhibit a wide range of non-verbal behaviors, process dialogs, and adapt to participants' actions. Moreover, the goal is to control the purpose and difficulty of social interactions, allowing the system to adapt to and train users with different abilities. To achieve this, we are advancing the following research:

1. **Interactive System**: Implementation of a chat-based dialog system with a system initiative and listening dialog (appropriate listening behavior).
2. **SST Scenarios/Steps** (Dialog Goal: Behavioral Change): (1) Setting the situation and goals: Setting typical social skill challenges; (2) Modeling: The trainer acts as a model and demonstrates the skills; (3) Role-play: The user engages in role-playing; (4) Feedback: The trainer provides feedback (with positive feedback here); (5) Homework: The trainer assigns small homework tasks for the user to carry out in everyday social interactions.
3. **CBT Scenarios/Steps** (Dialog Goal: Changing Negative Emotions): (1) Situation/Trigger: Describing the situation that led to the user's negative emotions; (2) Emotions: Organizing what the user feels; (3) Unhelpful Thoughts: Identifying the false beliefs or thought patterns behind the user's emotions; (4) Evidence: Finding evidence that supports the user's false beliefs; (5) Challenging these thoughts: Finding facts that contradict the user's unhelpful thoughts; (6) Alternative/More Balanced Beliefs: Helping the user understand healthier ways of thinking; (7) Results: Reassessing the user's emotions and feelings.

This research project was initiated in October 2019 as a Japan-France international joint ANR-CREST research project. On the Japanese side, it involves Nara Institute of Science and Technology, Osaka University, and Nara Medical University. On the French side, it involves CNRS-ISIR (Institut des Systèmes Intelligents et de Robotique) and CNRS-LISN (Laboratoire Interdisciplinaire des Sciences du Numérique). The SST training system results from joint research between Nara Institute of Science and Technology and Nara Medical University, while the CBT component is based on joint research between Nara Institute of Science and Technology and Osaka University. The virtual agent platform uses a system previously developed by CNRS-ISIR. This book highlights the research outcomes of this project.

This research has been conducted with support from the Japan Science and Technology Agency (JST) CREST program on the Japanese side and the Agence Nationale de la Recherche (ANR) on the French side, starting in October 2019 and lasting approximately five years.

Social Skills Theoretical Framework

Jennifer Hamet Bagnou, Elise Prigent, Jean-Claude Martin, and Céline Clavel

Abstract This chapter examines various psychological approaches that have sought to understand and conceptualize social competence and social skills. We explore several theoretical models that attempt to define the key notions surrounding this competence, highlighting the distinction between social skills, which are observable and acquired, and social competence, which is more global and multidimensional. These models provide frameworks for analyzing social adaptation, performance in specific tasks, and social skills, while considering contextual influences and the evaluation by others in assessing social effectiveness.

1 Introduction

Humans are characterized by profound social interdependence, as highlighted by Aristotle when he declared that "Man is a social animal" [1]. At the core of the network of interactions, relationships, and structures that form the foundation of societal life lies social competence—a set of interpersonal abilities that enable us to interact effectively and harmoniously with others. Despite universal recognition of the importance of social competence, researchers still struggle to agree on a unified and clear definition. Often intertwined with "social skills" and even used interchangeably in the literature, these two notions remain closely related but conceptually distinct. This terminological ambiguity, fueled by English translations favoring the term "skill" over "competence," is not merely academic but has significant theoretical and practical implications for research, education, and clinical intervention [2, 3].

Social skill is generally considered the requisite ability that enables a social response [4, 5]. It can encompass so-called molecular skills like eye contact and tone of voice, as well as more molar and global skill sets like social problem-solving [4, 6–8]. Social skills may be already acquired or can be trained, and it is used to modify social performance to meet the changing demands of tasks [4, 6, 7].

J. Hamet Bagnou (✉) · E. Prigent · J.-C. Martin · C. Clavel
Interdisciplinary Laboratory of Digital Sciences (LISN), Cognition, Perception and Uses Team, CNRS, Université Paris Saclay, Orsay, France
e-mail: hamet@lisn.fr

S. Nakamura (ed.), *Multimodal Interaction Technologies for Training Affective Social Skills*, https://doi.org/10.1007/978-981-96-1313-7_2

Most existing definitions of *social competence* refer to effectiveness, focus on individual behavior (rather than on dyads or groups), and consider the influence of situational context [4, 9]. Despite commonalities among various definitions, what constitutes socially competent behavior remains somewhat difficult to determine, mainly because the competent response is relative (judgment by others) and depends on multiple contextual factors. The most contemporary models consider social competence to be at a very global level, multidimensional and to encompass social adaptation, social performance, and social skills. Social adaptation assesses the ability to achieve social goals in accordance with societal and age-related expectations. Social performance measures effectiveness in specific social tasks. Social skills combine overt behaviors and sociocognitive processes to generate contextual social performances [4, 6, 8].

2 Historical Background and Definitions

The foundations for understanding social competence can be traced back to the pioneering work of Thorndike and other researchers in the field of *social intelligence* [10–13]. Thorndike formulated the idea of intelligence comprising three facets: verbal, numerical, and conceptual intelligence; mechanical and material intelligence; and social intelligence [10]. The latter component, termed social intelligence, was described as "the ability to understand and manage human interactions wisely" [10, 14]. Similarly, Hunt [15] characterized "social intelligence" as "the faculty to collaborate harmoniously with others." Vernon [16] further elaborated by proposing a more detailed definition of social intelligence, describing it as "the capacity to interact effectively with individuals in general, master social codes, navigate social environments with ease, understand social issues, be receptive to signals emitted by others within a group, and grasp the emotional nuances and underlying personalities of strangers."

Wechsler's contribution rekindled interest in social intelligence, which he explored through a subtest of the Wechsler Adult Intelligence Scale (WAIS), assessing the understanding of social situations via images [17]. However, after two decades of testing, Wechsler [18] postulated that social intelligence might not be a distinct entity from general intelligence but rather a manifestation of it applied to social situations.

The renewed debate by Guilford and his colleagues on behavioral intelligence in the 1960s, as well as on the assessment of empathy, expanded the conception of intelligence to encompass emotional intelligence, defined as the ability to perceive, express, integrate, understand, and regulate emotions [19–21].

While social intelligence refers to the cognitive ability to understand and manage human interactions wisely, the concept of social competence builds on this by encompassing not only understanding but also the ability to effectively manage interactions and influence interpersonal responses. This shift from social intelligence to social competence marks a significant conceptual evolution, where competencies become observable behaviors in real-world social interactions.

White [22] and Weinstein [23] laid the groundwork for modern definitions of social competence, emphasizing the effectiveness of interaction with the environment and the ability to manipulate interpersonal responses.

Zigler and Trickett [24] then attempted to define social competence using a dual approach that reflects the child's success in meeting social expectations and self-realization or personal development. Their definition included measures of physical health and well-being, formal cognitive abilities, outcomes, motivational and emotional variables.

The field of social competence was further enriched with definitions such as that of Rubin and Rose-Krasnor [8, 25], considering social competence as the ability to achieve personal goals while maintaining positive relationships in various social contexts.

It was McFall [26] who made a significant advance by differentiating social skills from social competence. According to him, social skills are necessary but not sufficient for adequate competence in social tasks—a crucial distinction for subsequent social assessments [4]. Later, Gresham [27] defined social competence as an evaluative term based on others' judgments in social situations.

In addition to these conceptualizations of social competence that include effectiveness in social interactions as a central aspect, some researchers consider social competence primarily in terms of a set of desirable social skills [6, 27–31]. Social skills are then defined as the ability to interact with others in a given social context in an appropriate manner (e.g., interacting in a formal meeting versus during a coffee break between colleagues), which is socially acceptable or valued and at the same time personally beneficial, mutually beneficial, or primarily beneficial to others [32, 33]. Besides considering social competence from the perspective of social skills, research has also viewed social competence in terms of *social outcomes*. The social outcomes perspective includes being effective in achieving one's *social goals*. Social goals, according to Pervin [34], are the objectives an individual attempts to achieve in interactions with others.

This brief history of social competence summarized above shows us that more than a century after Thorndike's first definition [11], there still seems to be no consensus on what constitutes social competence. Indeed, depending on research objectives, epistemological nuances, and practical constraints, certain aspects of social functioning may be more important than others. Greenspan [35], e.g., noted that operational definitions of social competence differ depending on whether the focus is on outcomes, underlying cognitive skills, or observable content associated with social competence [6]. Many research articles in the field of social competence report a lack of an accepted conceptual definition for the term [4, 10, 29, 36, 37].

However, the past thirty years of research attest to the diversity, breadth, and richness of the concept of social competence, as well as its importance. We now understand that social competence is an organizational construct with interactional characteristics, context-dependent, performance-oriented, and goal-specific. Consequently, conceptual definitions of social competence can be characterized in terms of social skills, social interactions, social goals, or social outcomes.

3 Models of Social Competence

Given the multifaceted nature of social competence, several researchers have been developing different theoretical, measurement, and intervention models. Each of the models summarized below adopts a slightly different perspective. Considered together, they deepen our understanding of the concepts related to social competence. Grover and colleagues [4] classified models of social competence and social skills into four categories. Definitional models describe social skills and social competence and establish the relationships between the different concepts. Situational models focus on identifying so-called critical situations and encourage reflection on the social skills necessary in these situations. Process models attempt to facilitate the understanding of how different social skills can function together in a coordinated manner and thus form a system. Finally, key competence set models provide a holistic view of the wide range of competences that work in harmony to enable competent social interactions [4].

3.1 Definitional Models

Since the 1970s, research on social competence and the training of social competence has experienced significant growth. This increased interest has encouraged researchers to develop models defining these competences and to explore how they are related. These models aim to facilitate a consensus, thereby supporting theoretical and empirical development while guiding assessment and intervention practices.

Among the first to conceptualize these ideas, McFall [26], and Dodge and Murphy [28] distinguished social skills, social competence, and social tasks. McFall defines *social tasks* as forces that organize and direct behavior, illustrated by activities such as "having a conversation" or "developing an intimate relationship" [26]. These social tasks encompass different sub-levels of behaviors, like "making a friend," which may include actions such as "finding people with similar interests" and "initiating a shared social activity".

3.1.1 Three-Component Model of Social Competence

Cavell's three-component model of social competence proposes an integrative structure composed of three hierarchical levels [6]. At the base, *social adjustment* is defined as the ability to achieve social goals appropriate to one's developmental stage (e.g., employment, relationship status, and peer acceptance). This dimension is influenced by societal and cultural norms [4, 6, 24, 38].

The intermediate level, associated with social performance or social functioning, concerns the individual's ability to navigate social situations by meeting socially valid criteria. According to Cavell, social performance is the degree to which an individual's responses to relevant situations meet socially acceptable standards [4, 26, 28, 39, 40]. Through this dimension, Cavell emphasizes the importance of considering social validity—that is, the societal value of behavior and its link to relevant social outcomes—to evaluate social performance.

The final level concerns specific social skills that enable an individual to behave competently in social tasks, such as eye contact, turn-taking in conversation, or more complex skills like problem-solving, including cognitive and emotional processes. In accordance with the social information processing models proposed by Dodge [28] and McFall [26], these component skills or processes allow a sequence of functions: stimulus encoding, decision-making, and response implementation. Also included under the term social skills are overt behaviors as well as cognitive social skills [28, 41] and emotional regulation [38].

To summarize, according to the three-component model, social competence is a multi-level construct with three sub-components: social adjustment, social performance, and social skills. Social adjustment is the extent to which important developmental goals are being achieved. Social performance, which is the adequacy of one's behavior within relevant social tasks, is a necessary but insufficient determinant of social adjustment. Finally, social skills are distinct abilities that are necessary but insufficient for producing effective social performance.

The three-level prism model of social competence by Rose-Krasnor [8] complements and expands Cavell's model [4, 42].

At the highest level (theoretical level), we find social competence. According to Rose-Krasnor, social competence is defined as effective interaction that meets developmental needs. Social competence is considered a transactional concept, meaning it is evaluated based on others' reactions as well as the situation itself [8, 42]. Like Cavell [6, 20], Rose-Krasnor emphasizes that gender, culture, and developmental stage influence social competence. Rose-Krasnor adds that social competence also depends on the individual's goals for the given social situation (e.g., during a job interview) [4]. The intermediate level (index level) represents specific indicators of social competence (e.g., sociometric status, relationship quality, social self-efficacy). These indices are organized into two groups: Self (the focus is on the individual's needs and perspectives; e.g., self-efficacy) and Others (the focus is on social connections; e.g., sociometric status, relationship quality). These indices constitute a "balance" between autonomy and interdependence [4]. Social competence is perceived as the ability to manage one's own needs while maintaining relationships with others. Finally, at the base of the prism is the skills/abilities level. This level includes the social, behavioral, emotional, cognitive, and motivational components of social competence. The skills level is considered fundamental because these abilities likely impact the indices at the level above [4].

3.1.2 Conclusion About the Three-Component Model of Social Competence

Definitional models present social competence as both a transactional and hierarchical concept. According to this approach, social competence is evaluated through others' reactions and the specifics of the situation, while being structured around three distinct levels. Although the terminology varies from one author to another, the underlying principles remain similar. Cavell, in his tripartite model, articulates social competence around adaptability to cultural and social norms, acceptable management of social situations, and specific skills that enhance social effectiveness. These competences include both cognitive abilities, such as causal inferences, and emotional abilities, like emotion regulation.

Rose-Krasnor defines social competence by its effectiveness in interactions, emphasizing the importance of balancing individual needs and those of others. She also introduces the concepts of personal motivation and goals specific to given situations.

The contributions of Cavell and Rose-Krasnor suggest that social skills are essential but not sufficient to ensure effective social competence, which requires a broader set of personal characteristics and motivations.

However, these models focus mainly on the conceptual framework of social competence, often neglecting direct contextual influences and the diversity of practical social skills. This limitation highlights a critical need to reevaluate definitional models to better integrate situational aspects, which are crucial for understanding and accurately assessing social competence in various environments.

3.2 Situational Models

Several definitions of social skills and social competence highlight the importance of the situation; however, few suggest methods for evaluating the significance of specific situations.

Situational models of social competence emphasize the crucial role of specific contexts in the assessment and development of social competence. According to this approach, social competence is not a static entity but rather a dynamic ability that evolves in response to the specific demands of each situation [4, 6–8, 43–46]. This theoretical framework allows us to understand social competence as a flexible adaptation to the various social environments encountered by an individual.

3.2.1 Behavioral Analysis Model of Goldfried and D'Zurilla

The behavioral analysis model of Goldfried and D'Zurilla [39] features a five-step process designed to operationalize and assess social competence. According to this model, an effective response is one that transforms the situation to render it non-problematic while maximizing positive consequences and minimizing negative ones. This definition allows for evaluating the degree of social competence by examining the potential impacts of each behavioral response in defined contexts, offering a spectrum of responses that can be evaluated incrementally.

3.2.2 Conclusion of the Situational Model

The situational model is focused on the evaluation of competences. It generates a measure of outcomes and does not take into account the underlying social skills, goals, and motivations that can promote competence [4].

One of the main advantages of this model is its ability to produce situation-specific measures that are directly relevant to specific groups of participants. This allows for a more precise and relevant assessment of social competence. However, the method heavily relies on consensus, which may limit the recognition of innovative or creative responses that do not conform to established norms.

Moreover, although the model is robust for competence evaluation, it does not dwell on the underlying social skills, goals, or motivations that facilitate social competence. This gap can be critical because understanding the underlying factors can enrich interventions aimed at improving social competence.

3.3 Process Models

Researchers argue that an intervention focused on cognitive and behavioral processes can be more effective than one centered solely on the development of isolated social skills, often referred to as "molecular" skills. Trower [47] emphasizes that fundamental social skills lie in the ability to generate appropriate behaviors that meet both the individual's personal objectives and situational demands. From this perspective, Trower's generative model of social skills [47] and the Social Information Processing (SIP) model by Crick & Dodge [48] and Dodge & Murphy [49] focus on the cognitive processes responsible for socially competent responses. These models provide an overview of how various social skills can interact within an integrated system, thereby identifying specific areas for assessment and intervention.

3.3.1 Social Information Processing (SIP) Model

The Social Information Processing (SIP) model developed by Dodge and colleagues describes a five-step cognitive sequence for social responses. The process begins with the decoding of important social cues, requiring particular vigilance to key social information [48]. The second step involves interpreting these cues to understand their meaning. For example, a stranger might bump into someone's coffee cup while passing on a sidewalk. The person who was bumped will use both relevant social cues (e.g., facial expressions, gestures, degree of sidewalk congestion) and personal memory (e.g., scanning past similar situations) to determine the stranger's intent (e.g., accidental or hostile). This is followed by a search for possible responses, where the individual rapidly evaluates different potential actions. The response decision constitutes the fourth step, selecting the best option among potential responses. Finally, the execution of the chosen response is implemented, and the effectiveness of this response is monitored to allow for adjustments if necessary. To be effective, the person must track the outcome of this response and be able to adapt the response if needed [48].

The SIP operates within a broader context of the specific social task demands, the individual's social goals, and memories of past experiences, all of which can influence decisions made at each step [4, 48]. Deficits can occur at any of the stages or at multiple levels. Moreover, as with other definitions of social competence, the evaluative judgment of other involved individuals determines whether the chosen behavior is socially competent.

McFall and colleagues [26, 41] developed a similar social information processing model articulated around three key phases: stimulus encoding, decision-making, and response enactment. This sequential model provides a structured framework for examining the cognitive processes underlying social interactions.

Encoding skills involve the reception, perception, and interpretation of stimuli related to the social task. Substantial research in this area has focused on how individuals perceive and interpret social information. Key variables include recognition and definition of social problems [50], identification of appropriate social goals [51], empathy and perspective-taking [52, 53], personal attributions and those made to others [54], as well as detection of intent cues [49]. These skills are essential for effectively navigating social interactions by providing a basis for subsequent adaptive responses.

Decision-making skills represent a phase of the process characterized by searching for, evaluating, and selecting possible responses. Response options are assessed based on their fit with the individual's behavioral repertoire and anticipated costs and benefits. Studies have examined various aspects of this skill, including the generation of alternative responses and decision-making [50], the ability to consider alternative consequences and outcomes [55], evaluations of self-efficacy and outcome expectancies[56, 57], and functional skills such as formulating and justifying actions and evaluating their impact on others [58].

Response enactment competence encompasses the planned execution of behaviors as well as the adjustment of these behaviors in response to received feedback. It integrates the representation of behavioral scenarios [59], self-regulation and behavioral planning [60], as well as self-instructions [61]. Manifest behaviors, whether verbal (instructions, questions, expressions of feelings) or non-verbal (eye contact, gestures, facial expressions), are also considered [47]. The importance of measuring specific skills, such as turn-taking management or eye contact usage, lies in their integration into a sequential approach. This approach allows not only for detecting shared variance between different skills but also for formulating hypotheses about the relationships between specific skills and predicting overall social performance by combining scores from various measures [6, 62].

3.3.2 Four-Dimensional Model

Most definitions of social competence have suggested that it involves the effectiveness of a person's functioning as an individual, in dyadic relationships, and in groups [63]. Rubin and Rose-Krasnor [5, 25] defined social competence as the ability to achieve personal goals in social interaction while simultaneously maintaining positive relationships with others over time and across situations. An important feature of this definition is the implicit recognition of the importance of individual and social goals.

Bukowski and colleagues [63] suggested an essential duality between self and others, placing the individual in a social context and a personal context. The definition by Rubin and Rose-Krasnor [25] highlights the complex goals individuals face as both individuals (satisfying personal objectives) and as group members (while maintaining positive relationships). Like Cavell and Rose-Krasnor, Yeates considers social competence as a transactional construct. From this perspective, social competence is also regarded as a developmental construct [5, 25].

Rubin, Bukowski, and Parker [63] suggest that the study of social competence can be guided in part by distinguishing several levels of social complexity: individuals, interactions, and relationships. People bring individual characteristics in their interactions with others (e.g., the ability to regulate emotions; the ability to predict the consequences of strategies chosen to achieve social goals, both for oneself and for others; thoughts and feelings concerning the individual's ability to succeed in the social world). Yeates et al. [5] suggest that these individual characteristics constitute individuals' social intelligence. In turn, people's social interactions also depend on individual characteristics and the behavior of those with whom they interact. Social interactions can be characterized as involving actions that bring individuals together (i.e., sociable and prosocial behaviors), actions that push people against each other (i.e., aggression), and actions that isolate individuals from one another (i.e., social withdrawal; [63]). Finally, interactions give rise to long-term relationships. Relationships are defined in part by the members and the quality of their interactions but have properties that are their own, such as closeness and commitment.

The contributions of factors related to the individual, behavior, situation, and evaluator are considered in the definition of social competence proposed by McFall [26] in a given situation. In their meta-analysis integrating theoretical, measurement, and intervention models of youth social competence, Dirks et al. [7] propose a four-dimensional model of social competence: the individual, the behavior, the situation, and the evaluator. In other words, knowing the individual in question, the situation in which the behavior was adopted, the chosen behavior, and the person evaluating the behavior would explain the greatest variability in a person's social functioning. In this model, Dirks revisits the previously discussed models—the definitional model and the situational model—while adding additional predictors.

3.3.3 Conclusion of Process Models

Process models define social competence as a set of appropriate behaviors that meet the individual's social goals and situational demands. This definition underscores several points:

- The behavior must be judged by relevant individuals to be considered competent (or not).
- The behavior occurs within a specific social situation.
- The behavior must meet social goals and norms.
- The behavior is performed by a specific individual (with their endogenous and exogenous characteristics).

These models draw inspiration from the three-component structure of the definitional models of Cavell [6] and Rose-Krasnor [8], to which they add the processes impacting a skill to render it competent or not. They develop methods of assessment and intervention (e.g., Yeates [5]). However, they only partly consider other non-cognitive factors (e.g., behavioral factors) that can affect response capacity.

3.4 Social Skills Sets Model

It is important to consider models that identify sets of essential social skills for a socially competent response. Social skills are always contextual, and even models based on sets of competences assume that an agreed-upon goal of social performance is established. These models play a crucial role as they detail specific domains for assessment and intervention.

3.4.1 Definitions and Historical Background

Extensive research is required to identify the sets of social skills most critical for social functioning. McFall [26], in one of the earliest models of this type, distinguished three systems of social skills: physiological, cognitive, and overt behavioral. According to McFall, physiological skills include sensory processes and those related to biological regulation and control.

Cognitive skills are primarily viewed through the lens of information processing, as described above in the section on process models. McFall also highlights the importance of verbal and non-verbal motor competences as essential components of social skills.

Subsequent models have enriched and expanded upon the three domains highlighted by McFall [26]. For example, Felner, Lease, and Phillips [64] review the literature on social skills and proposed a four-part model, identifying behavioral and cognitive competences as crucial. These researchers extend McFall's framework by integrating cultural knowledge about social norms and decision-making as fundamental cognitive competences. They also emphasize the importance of emotional regulation and emotional competence, encompassing the management of intense negative emotions and the development of positive affective bonds. Additionally, they recognize that motivation and expectations play a determining role in our social behaviors.

Over time, key competence set models have become more inclusive and contextually adaptive. Spence [65] introduces a new model that takes into account behavioral, cognitive, emotional, and environmental factors. This model is noteworthy for its inclusion of specific environmental influences that can affect social skills. Deficits can appear in one or more domains, necessitating a multisectoral evaluation to design an effective intervention. Milligan and colleagues [66] distilled the literature on social skills into three target domains: behavioral, cognitive, and emotional, while integrating knowledge about neuropsychological factors influencing these skills, such as attentional control and executive functioning. The authors emphasize that competences in each domain often interact dynamically with those in other domains, illustrating the complexity and interdependence of the processes involved in social competence.

3.4.2 Riggio's Model

Riggio [67] proposes a general framework for several fundamental social skills of social competence and the construction of a self-assessment tool to measure them. His definition of basic social skills assumes that they are acquired social abilities and strategies. A social skill is defined by the particular social and cultural norms that govern interpersonal communication [67]. According to Riggio et al. [67], basic social skills play an important role in managing complex social behaviors (e.g., empathy, emotional intelligence, the ability to communicate one's thoughts or feelings, etc.). This model considers social skills as a relatively stable and enduring personality trait (trait model).

Riggio's theory stems from multidisciplinary research on social and interpersonal competence but derives more directly from psychologists' attempts to measure individual differences in non-verbal communication skills [68–72]. Each of these research avenues primarily addresses a distinct dimension of communication aptitude: communication sensitivity, communication expressiveness, and communication monitoring or control.

The skills involved in sending and receiving information are represented in the basic social skills of expressiveness and sensitivity. Riggio [69], in his study on the assessment of basic social skills, was primarily interested in the communication of non-verbal messages, particularly the sending and receiving of emotional expressions. Thus, the first four social skills in this article are called: emotional expressiveness, emotional sensitivity, social expressiveness, and social sensitivity. Although two of these dimensions are called emotional expressiveness and emotional sensitivity, they encompass more than just the ability to communicate emotions.

Emotional expressiveness involves the ability to communicate affect, attitudes, and status. Emotional sensitivity is the ability to decode others' emotions, beliefs, or attitudes and the dominance cues of their status. Social expressiveness includes verbal expressive ability, verbal fluency, and the capacity to engage in conversations. The ability to receive and understand verbal messages, along with knowledge and concern for social rules and norms, are central elements of social sensitivity [69]. Two other skills pertain to communication control. The skill of emotional control is the ability to regulate emotional communications and non-verbal displays. Social control includes the ability to play a role, regulate verbal behavior, and self-presentation skills.

In summary, there are six dimensions of social skills involving the ability to send, receive, and control communication in two distinct domains: the emotional-non-verbal domain and the social-verbal domain. It is important to mention that these dimensions of basic competences are intended to represent a general breakdown of social communication skills. This is by no means an exhaustive list. We will also see, in the section entitled "Individual Differences Impacting Social Competence," that these dimensions can give rise to different types of profiles and thus contribute to the variance in social competence.

3.4.3 Grover's Model

Grover et al. define and present a model comprising four domains of social skills: communication, cognitive skills, emotion, and problem-solving ability. These domains were chosen "based on their links with models and their common inclusion in social skills interventions" [4]. Below, we detail the four domains of social skills deemed essential for effective social performance.

Communication occurs when a message from one person, the sender, modifies the behavior of another person, the receiver [4]. Communication is thus at the heart of interpersonal interactions. It includes verbal and non-verbal elements that interact to facilitate mutual understanding between the sender and the receiver. Verbal communication primarily involves the use of language, while non-verbal communication includes voice qualities such as rhythm, tone, or intonation patterns; eye contact; gestures; body language or posture; touch; proxemics (i.e., the use and understanding of space); and facial expressions [73].

Emotion regulation refers to an individual's efforts to influence the type, intensity, timing, and expression of her emotional experience [4]. These efforts can occur automatically or be conscious and intentional. Emotion regulation strategies focused on antecedents aim to modify the emotional response before it occurs. For example, an individual might change their thoughts about a situation (cognitive change), avoid a situation or person that elicits strong emotion (situation selection), or focus their attention on more pleasant aspects of a situation (attentional deployment). Response-focused strategies target emotional reactions already engaged and are called response modulation strategies. For example, an individual might try to suppress the emotional experience or modify the behavioral expression of the emotion. Disruption of emotions could negatively impact the acquisition or performance of social skills, or both, and thus influence the presence or quality of social relationships.

As suggested by the process and skills models described above, several cognitive factors contribute to social competence. Cognitive social skills refer to the knowledge, thoughts, and reasoning involved in social interactions. For example, informational knowledge helps individuals understand and predict each person's role and the actions that may be necessary in a specific social context. Social Information Processing (SIP; previously discussed) involves several steps, including encoding social cues, interpreting these cues, clarifying social goals, generating responses, making response decisions, and enacting behavior [48]. Attributions or beliefs concerning events and other factors also influence social behavior. Other cognitive skills that impact social functioning include Theory of Mind (ToM), which influences the interpretation or understanding of others' emotions and behaviors. ToM reflects the ability to attribute various mental states (i.e., beliefs, desires, emotions) to others and to recognize that these mental states may differ from one's own [4, 66]. The processing of social and cognitive information is also influenced by basic neuropsychological abilities involving aspects of attention, processing speed, executive functions, and visuospatial processing [4, 66].

Emotional disorders, such as social anxiety and depression, are characterized by cognitive biases and negative patterns that influence SIP. As greater attention is paid by these individuals to negative information and negative attributions about peers' behaviors, this contributes to more negative social interactions [4]. Individuals with deficits in basic neuropsychological abilities, such as those with Attention Deficit Hyperactivity Disorder (ADHD), also struggle to form and maintain friendships, complete their studies or work, and are more exposed to other internalizing and externalizing problems [66].

Several models of social competence described in the previous sections refer to the ability to adapt and respond to a variety of social situations. The skill of social problem-solving is the process by which individuals identify effective and adaptive responses to everyday life problems [39]. Problems are real dilemmas (social or otherwise) that may involve personal, interpersonal, or broader social difficulties (e.g., job loss, managing a conflict with a peer, or experiencing discrimination). When problems arise without an obvious solution, individuals use their social problem-solving skills to find solutions that maximize positive consequences and minimize negative consequences. The individual must consider his personal goals and the social context, as well as short- and long-term outcomes, to identify the most adaptive solution. Social problem-solving begins with a general problem orientation, which refers to an individual's typical attitude or schema activated in response to problems [74]. An adaptive or positive problem orientation involves the ability to recognize problems, acceptance of problems as an inherent aspect of daily life, and belief in one's ability to solve the problem [75]. Conversely, a maladaptive or negative problem orientation involves perceiving problems as unsolvable, doubting one's ability to solve the problem, and frustration or intolerance toward a problem. Beyond the general problem orientation, the social problem-solving process involves specific skills: (a) problem definition and formulation, (b) generation of alternatives, (c) decision-making, and (d) solution implementation and verification [50]. These components are not necessarily a sequential process but overlap or repeat until a solution is successful. Difficulty in implementing effective social problem-solving skills impacts adaptive functioning in children [18, 63], adults [18, 64], and the elderly [18, 65].

3.4.4 Conclusion About the Social Skill Sets Models

The key social skills models aim to enumerate basic social skills—that is, those that serve as starting points for other skills and are fundamental for being socially competent. Thus, although not all social skills can be identified and labeled, a significant number of them, exhibiting different levels of complexity, have been clearly defined and proven important (Grover et al., 2020).

According to Riggio, social skill is a relatively stable and enduring personality trait. It is defined by the particular social and cultural norms that govern interpersonal communication. Riggio's model asserts that good social skills involve abilities to encode, decode, and control one's emotions and sociability [67]. Accordingly, Riggio defined six essential social skills for interpersonal communication: emotional expressiveness, emotional sensitivity, and emotional control in the context of verbal communication, and the same for non-verbal communication. However, this model is limited to interpersonal communication skills and does not consider cognitive skills that can influence social performance [67].

Each of the subsequent models presents basic social skills that can be either similar or complementary. The model proposed by Grover appears to be the most comprehensive among them. Indeed, Grover and his collaborators, on both theoretical and practical grounds, propose communication skills, emotion regulation, cognitive skills, and social problem-solving as the basic social skills [4].

Social skills sets models offer a definite advantage in developing intervention strategies or in research. They propose sets of skills that can be directly targeted by intervention for training them. However, these models should not be used alone. Indeed, they emphasize the behavioral dimension while omitting the importance of the situation in which the behavior occurred, the individual executing the behavior, and the people who judge this behavior [4].

4 Conclusion

This chapter highlights the complexity and diversity of approaches to the notions of social competence and social skills. Over the past decades, numerous authors have underscored the multiplicity of definitions and the lack of consensus surrounding social competence, thus complicating the harmonization of evaluative and intervention approaches [4, 5, 7, 10, 62].

We identified a consensus around the notion of effectiveness in social interaction, which heavily depends on context and evaluation by others. Building on theories established by figures such as Cavell, Rose-Krasnor, and Yeates, we developed an integrative and heuristic model of social competence [4, 6]. This model describes social competence as a multidimensional entity, encompassing social adaptation, social performance, and social skills [4, 8]. Social adaptation measures the ability to achieve social goals appropriate to one's age and societal expectations; social performance evaluates effectiveness in specific social tasks; and social skills combine overt behaviors and sociocognitive processes to generate contextual performances.

To be considered socially competent, it is essential that an individual uses social skills in a way that respects social norms and appropriately responds to the emotions and thoughts of others. Each of these skills can be observed at the behavioral level. However, social interactions are complex, and it is rare for a single social behavior to be adopted in isolation. It is crucial to pay attention to the contextual, verbal, and non-verbal cues of social partners and to integrate this information with prior experiences and knowledge to develop an appropriate respons [4, 66].

References

1. P. Pellegrin, *Aristote Les Politiques*. https://editions.flammarion.com/les-politiques/9782081358775. Accessed 22 Apr 2024
2. J. Hughes, Assessment of social skills: sociometric and behavioral approaches, in *Handbook of psychological and educational assessment of children*, (1990), pp. 423–444
3. K. Renk, V. Phares, Cross-informant ratings of social competence in children and adolescents. Clin. Psychol. Rev. **24**(2), 239–254 (2004). https://doi.org/10.1016/j.cpr.2004.01.004
4. R.L. Grover, D.W. Nangle, M. Buffie, and L.A. Andrews, Defining social skills, in *Social Skills Across the Life Span*, (Elsevier, 2020), pp. 3–24. https://doi.org/10.1016/B978-0-12-817752-5.00001-9
5. K.O. Yeates et al., Social outcomes in childhood brain disorder: a heuristic integration of social neuroscience and developmental psychology. Psychol. Bull. **133**(3), 535–556 (2007). https://doi.org/10.1037/0033-2909.133.3.535
6. T. Cavell, Social adjustment, social performance, and social skills: a tri-component model of social competence. J. Clin. Child Adolesc. Psychol. **19**(2), 111–122 (1990). https://doi.org/10.1207/s15374424jccp1902_2
7. M.A. Dirks, T.A. Treat, V.R. Weersing, The situation specificity of youth responses to peer provocation. J. Clin. Child Adolesc. Psychol. **36**(4), 621–628 (2007). https://doi.org/10.1080/15374410701662758
8. L. Rose-Krasnor, The nature of social competence: a theoretical review. Soc. Dev. **6**(1), 111–135 (1997). https://doi.org/10.1111/j.1467-9507.1997.tb00097.x
9. D.W. Nangle, R.L. Grover, L.J. Holleb, M. Cassano, J. Fales, Defining Competence and Identifying Target Skills, in *Practitioner's Guide to Empirically Based Measures of Social Skills*, eds. D.W. Nangle, D.J. Hansen, C.A. Erdley, P.J. Norton (New York, NY: Springer, 2010), pp. 3–19. https://doi.org/10.1007/978-1-4419-0609-0_1
10. G.K. Pavliga, *Toward a Conceptual Definition for Social Competence an Exploratory Study*, (University of Akron, 2008)
11. E.L. Thorndike, The reliability and significance of tests of intelligence. J. Educ. Psychol. **11**(5), 284–287 (1920). https://doi.org/10.1037/h0074443

12. R.L. Thorndike, Factor analysis of social and abstract intelligence. J. Educ. Psychol. **27**(3), 231–233 (1936). https://doi.org/10.1037/h0059840
13. R.L. Thorndike, S. Stein, An evaluation of the attempts to measure social intelligence. Psychol. Bull. **34**(5), 275–285 (1937). https://doi.org/10.1037/h0053850
14. K.S. Law, C.-S. Wong, L.J. Song, The construct and criterion validity of emotional intelligence and its potential utility for management studies. J. Appl. Psychol. **89**(3), 483–496 (2004). https://doi.org/10.1037/0021-9010.89.3.483
15. T. Hunt, The measurement of social intelligence. J. Appl. Psychol. **12**(3), 317–334 (1928). https://doi.org/10.1037/h0075832
16. P.E. Vernon, Some characteristics of the good judge of personality. J. Soc. Psychol. **4**, 42–58 (1933). https://doi.org/10.1080/00224545.1933.9921556
17. D. Wechsler, *Wechsler Intelligence Scale for Children*, (Oxford, England: The Psychological Corp., 1949), p. 113
18. D. Wechsler, The Measurement and appraisal of adult intelligence. Acad. Med. **33**(9), 706 (1958)
19. R.B. Gunderman, Emotional intelligence. J. Am. Coll. Radiol. **8**(5), 298–299 (2011). https://doi.org/10.1016/j.jacr.2011.02.007
20. J.D. Mayer, P. Salovey, D.R. Caruso, Emotional Intelligence: theory, findings, and implications. Psychol. Inq. **15**(3), 197–215 (2004)
21. J.D. Mayer, G. Geher, Emotional intelligence and the identification of emotion. Intelligence **22**(2), 89–113 (1996). https://doi.org/10.1016/S0160-2896(96)90011-2
22. R.W. White, Motivation reconsidered: The concept of competence. Psychol. Rev. **66**(5), 297–333 (1959). https://doi.org/10.1037/h0040934
23. B.A. Weinstein, The development of interpersonal competence, 1969. https://www.semanticscholar.org/paper/The-development-of-interpersonal-competence-Weinstein/673c18d76696337880 68fc2d7339e9d176b91c5b. Accessed: 22 Apr 2024
24. E. Zigler, P.K. Trickett, IQ, social competence, and evaluation of early childhood intervention programs. Am. Psychol. **33**(9), 789–798 (1978). https://doi.org/10.1037/0003-066X.33.9.789
25. K. H. Rubin, L. Rose-Krasnor, Interpersonal problem solving and social competence in children, in *Handbook of social development: A lifespan perspective, Perspectives in developmental psychology*, (New York, NY, US: Plenum Press, 1992), pp. 283–323. https://doi.org/10.1007/978-1-4899-0694-6_12
26. R.M. McFall, A review and reformulation of the concept of social skills. Behav. Assess. **4**(1), 1–33 (1982). https://doi.org/10.1007/BF01321377
27. F.M. Gresham, Conceptual and definitional issues in the assessment of children's social skills: Implications for classification and training. J. Clin. Child Psychol. **15**(1), 3–15 (1986). https://doi.org/10.1207/s15374424jccp1501_1
28. K.A. Dodge, G.S. Pettit, C.L. McClaskey, M.M. Brown, J.M. Gottman, Social competence in children. Monogr. Soc. Res. Child Dev. **51**(2), i–85 (1986). https://doi.org/10.2307/1165906
29. J.A. Hubbard, J.D. Coie, Emotional correlates of social competence in children's peer relationships. Merrill-Palmer Q. **40**(1), 1–20 (1994)
30. J. Mize, G.W. Ladd, A cognitive-social learning approach to social skill training with low-status preschool children. Dev. Psychol. **26**(3), 388–397 (1990). https://doi.org/10.1037/0012-1649.26.3.388
31. E. Waters, L.A. Sroufe, Social competence as a developmental construct. Dev. Rev. **3**(1), 79–97 (1983). https://doi.org/10.1016/0273-2297(83)90010-2
32. P. Butcher, Social Skills in Interpersonal Communication. Ed. By Owen Hargie, *Christine Saunders and David Dickson.* (London: Croom Helm. 1981), pp 198. £11.95, £5.95 (paperback). Br. J. Psychiatry, **139**(2), p. 176 (1981), https://doi.org/10.1192/S0007125000133549.
33. O. Hargie, C. Saunders, D. Dickson, *Social Skills in Interpersonal Communication.* (Psychology Press, 1994)
34. L.A. Pervin, Goal concepts in personality and social psychology: A historical introduction, in *Goal concepts in personality and social psychology*, (Hillsdale, NJ, US: Lawrence Erlbaum Associates, Inc, 1989), pp. 1–17

35. S. Greenspan, Defining childhood social competence: a proposed working model. Adv. Spec. Educ. **3**, 1–39 (1981)
36. S.W. Smith, P.C. Travis, Conducting social competence research: considering conceptual frameworks. Behav. Disord. **26**(4), 360–369 (2001). https://doi.org/10.1177/019874290102600408
37. A. Zsolnai, Relationship between children's social competence, learning motivation and school achievement. Educ. Psychol. **22**(3), 317–329 (2002). https://doi.org/10.1080/01443410220138548
38. M.E. Ford, Social cognition and social competence in adolescence. Dev. Psychol. **18**(3), 323–340 (1982). https://doi.org/10.1037/0012-1649.18.3.323
39. M.R. Goldfried, T.J. D'Zurilla, A Behavioral-Analytic Model for Assessing Competence1 1The preparation of this paper was supported by Research Grant MH-15044 from the United States Public Health Service, National Institute of Mental Health. The authors are grateful to Anita P. Goldfried, Ronald N. Kent, David M. Pomeranz, and Charles D. Spielberger for their comments on an earlier version of the manuscript," in *Current Topics in Clinical and Community Psychology*, vol. 1, ed. C.D. Spielberger, (Elsevier, 1969), pp. 151–196. https://doi.org/10.1016/B978-1-4831-9972-6.50009-3
40. H. Hops, Children's social competence and skill: current research practices and future directions. Behav. Ther. **14**(1), 3–18 (1983). https://doi.org/10.1016/S0005-7894(83)80084-7
41. D.G. Schlundt, R.M. McFall, Classifying social situations: a comparison of five methods. Behav. Assess. **9**(1), 21–42 (1987)
42. M.R. Persich, M.D. Robinson, Five approaches to understanding interpersonal competence: a review and integration. Rev. Gen. Psychol. **26**(4), 464–486 (2022). https://doi.org/10.1177/10892680221085507
43. T.A. Cavell, M.L. Kelley, The checklist of adolescent problem situations. J. Clin. Child Psychol. **23**(3), 226–238 (1994). https://doi.org/10.1207/s15374424jccp2303_1
44. M.L. Combs, D.A. Slaby, Social-Skills training with children, in *Advances in Clinical Child Psychology*, eds. B.B. Lahey, A.E. Kazdin, (Boston, MA: Springer US, 1977), pp. 161–201. https://doi.org/10.1007/978-1-4613-9799-1_5
45. D.L. DuBois, R.D. Felner, The quadripartite model of social competence: Theory and applications to clinical intervention, in *Cognitive therapy with children and adolescents: A casebook for clinical practice*, (New York, NY, US: The Guilford Press, 1996), pp. 124–152
46. C.A. Erdley, S.R. Asher, A social goals perspective on children's social competence. J. Emot. Behav. Disord. **7**(3), 156–167 (1999). https://doi.org/10.1177/106342669900700304
47. P. Trower, Situational analysis of the components and processes of behavior of socially skilled and unskilled patients. J. Consult. Clin. Psychol. **48**(3), 327–339 (1980). https://doi.org/10.1037/0022-006X.48.3.327
48. N.R. Crick, K.A. Dodge, A review and reformulation of social information-processing mechanisms in children's social adjustment. Psychol. Bull. **115**(1), 74–101 (1994). https://doi.org/10.1037/0033-2909.115.1.74
49. K.A. Dodge, R.R. Murphy, The assessment of social competence in adolescents. Adv. Child Behav. Anal. Ther. **3**, 61–96 (1984)
50. T.J. D'Zurilla, M.R. Goldfried, Problem solving and behavior modification. J. Abnorm. Psychol. **78**(1), 107–126 (1971). https://doi.org/10.1037/h0031360
51. P.D. Renshaw, S.R. Asher, Children's goals and strategies for social interaction. Merrill-Palmer Q. **29**(3), 353–374 (1983)
52. M.J. Chandler, Egocentrism and antisocial behavior: the assessment and training of social perspective-taking skills. Dev. Psychol. **9**(3), 326–332 (1973). https://doi.org/10.1037/h0034974
53. R.L. Selman, *The growth of interpersonal understanding: Developmental and clinical analyses*. (Academy Press, 1980), https://ixtheo.de/Record/023756276. Accessed 01 Oct 2024
54. C.S. Dweck and E.L. Leggett, A social-cognitive approach to motivation and personality, *Motiv. Personal*, p. 18

55. M.B. Shure, G. Spivack, The problem-solving approach to adjustment: a competency-building model of primary prevention. Prev. Hum. Serv. **1**(1–2), 87–103 (1981). https://doi.org/10.1300/J293v01n01_06
56. A. Bandura, Self-efficacy: toward a unifying theory of behavioral change. Psychol. Rev. **84**(2), 191–215 (1977). https://doi.org/10.1037/0033-295X.84.2.191
57. V.A. Wheeler, G.W. Ladd, Assessment of children's self-efficacy for social interactions with peers. Dev. Psychol. **18**(6), 795–805 (1982). https://doi.org/10.1037/0012-1649.18.6.795
58. R.L. Selman, W. Beardslee, L.H. Schultz, M. Krupa, D. Podorefsky, Assessing adolescent interpersonal negotiation strategies: toward the integration of structural and functional models. Dev. Psychol. **22**(4), 450–459 (1986). https://doi.org/10.1037/0012-1649.22.4.450
59. R.P. Abelson, Script processing in attitude formation and decision making, in *Cognition and social behavior*, (Oxford, England: Lawrence Erlbaum, 1976), pp. xiii, 290–xiii, 290
60. W. Mischel, Convergences and challenges in the search for consistency. Am. Psychol. **39**(4), 351–364 (1984). https://doi.org/10.1037/0003-066X.39.4.351
61. D.H. Meichenbaum, J. Goodman, Training impulsive children to talk to themselves: a means of developing self-control. J. Abnorm. Psychol. **77**(2), 115–126 (1971). https://doi.org/10.1037/h0030773
62. K.A. Dodge, Attributional bias in aggressive children, in *Advances in cognitive-behavioral research and therapy,* in Advances in cognitive-behavioral research and therapy, vol. 4, (San Diego, CA, US: Academic Press, 1985), pp. 73–110. https://doi.org/10.1016/B978-0-12-010604-2.50009-4
63. K.H. Rubin, W.M. Bukowski, J.G. Parker, Peer Interactions, Relationships, and Groups, in *Handbook of child psychology: Social, emotional, and personality development,* vol. 3, 6th ed. (Hoboken, NJ, US: Wiley, 2006), pp. 571–645
64. R.D. Felner, R.S. Phillips, D. DuBois, A.M. Lease, Ecological interventions and the process of change for prevention: wedding theory and research to implementation in real world settings. Am. J. Community Psychol. **19**(3), 379–387 (1991)
65. S.H. Spence, Social skills training with children and young people: theory, evidence and practice: therapy matters: social skills training. Child Adolesc. Ment. Health **8**(2), 84–96 (2003). https://doi.org/10.1111/1475-3588.00051
66. K. Milligan, A. Sibalis, A. Morgan, M. Phillips, Social Competence: Consideration of Behavioral, Cognitive, and Emotional Factors, in *Handbook of Childhood Psychopathology and Developmental Disabilities Treatment*, ed. By J.L. Matson, in *Autism and Child Psychopathology Series*, (Cham: Springer International Publishing, 2017), pp. 301–320. https://doi.org/10.1007/978-3-319-71210-9_18
67. R.E. Riggio, B. Throckmorton, S. DePaola, Social skills and self-esteem. Personal. Individ. Differ. **11**(8), 799–804 (1990). https://doi.org/10.1016/0191-8869(90)90188-W
68. R. Rosenthal, The file drawer problem and tolerance for null results. Psychol. Bull. **86**(3), 638–641 (1979). https://doi.org/10.1037/0033-2909.86.3.638
69. R.E. Riggio, Assessment of basic social skills. J. Pers. Soc. Psychol. **51**(3), 649–660 (1986). https://doi.org/10.1037/0022-3514.51.3.649
70. H.S. Friedman, L.M. Prince, R.E. Riggio, M.R. DiMatteo, Understanding and assessing nonverbal expressiveness: the affective communication test. J. Pers. Soc. Psychol. **39**(2), 333–351 (1980). https://doi.org/10.1037/0022-3514.39.2.333
71. M. Snyder, Self-monitoring of expressive behavior. J. Pers. Soc. Psychol. **30**(4), 526–537 (1974). https://doi.org/10.1037/h0037039
72. R.D. Lennox, R.N. Wolfe, Revision of the Self-monitoring scale. J. Pers. Soc. Psychol. **46**(6), 1349–1364 (1984). https://doi.org/10.1037/0022-3514.46.6.1349
73. S. Duncan Jr., Nonverbal communication. Psychol. Bull. **72**(2), 118–137 (1969). https://doi.org/10.1037/h0027795
74. T.J. D'Zurilla, Problem-solving training for effective stress management and prevention. J. Cogn. Psychother. **4**(4), 327–354 (1990)
75. A. Maydeu-Olivares, T.J. D'Zurilla, A factor-analytic study of the social problem-solving Inventory: an integration of theory and data. Cogn. Ther. Res. **20**(2), 115–133 (1996). https://doi.org/10.1007/BF02228030

Theory of Social Skills Training (SST)

Mitsuhiro Uratani and Tsubasa Morimoto

Abstract Social skills training (SST) is a structured approach to improving how individuals interact with others. It focuses on developing specific skills that help people navigate interpersonal situations more effectively. SST is used for all ages, from children to adults, and is also used for people with psychiatric disorders, such as autism spectrum disorder (ASD) and schizophrenia, who have difficulty building interpersonal relationships. Previous studies have reported that SST is useful in improving social skills, including those of people with psychiatric disorders. However, SST requires multiple facilitators with specific expertise, making access to it difficult. To overcome such disadvantages, this study investigates the usefulness of automated SST-based technology. This chapter describes conventional SST for children and adults, as well as the type of SST used in this research.

1 Introduction

Social skills training SST is a treatment designed to help people develop the skills they need for daily life. SST has been used for more than 40 years to help people who struggle to lead a normal social life. SST primarily targets the acquisition of interpersonal skills, and it is used to overcome barriers to social life caused by a lack of interpersonal skills. SST has been widely employed with people who lack social and communication skills. Accordingly, SST has also been widely used among people with psychiatric disorders. Previous work has reported that SST can be useful in improving interpersonal communication skills. Various SST models have been applied across the lifespan, from children to elderly adults. In this research, we

M. Uratani (✉) · T. Morimoto
Department of Psychiatry, Nara Medical University, Kashihara, Japan
e-mail: ura-mitsu0121@naramed-u.ac.jp

T. Morimoto
e-mail: tsubasa@naramed-u.ac.jp

M. Uratani
Manyo Clinic, Kashihara, Japan

S. Nakamura (ed.), *Multimodal Interaction Technologies for Training Affective Social Skills*, https://doi.org/10.1007/978-981-96-1313-7_3

conducted SST for typically developing (TD) children and children with autism spectrum disorder (ASD), as well as SST for healthy control (HC) adults and adults with schizophrenia or ASD. We also conducted automated SST using virtual agents. In this chapter, we illustrate the theory of SST for adults and for children by presenting our research as an example. In addition, we discuss the problems of human–human SST and the need for automated SST-based technology.

2 Social Skills Training (SST) for Adults

SST has been developed as a method that views interpersonal behavior disorders from the perspective of life skills, and it systematically works on both cognitive and behavioral skills to improve them. SST evolved from assertiveness training, which was conducted for people with interpersonal challenges such as shyness, and it has a long history comparable to psychoeducational or behavioral therapy. As a comprehensive treatment package, SST was developed by R.P. Liberman et al. in the 1970s, later expanded to include chronic psychiatric disorders, and widely adopted in Europe and the United States. In Japan, the first visit to the country by Liberman in 1988 marked the beginning of a full-scale spread of SST there. Currently, SST is integrated with other therapies and practiced in various fields such as health, medicine, welfare, rehabilitation, and industry, targeting not only schizophrenia but also various psychiatric disorders [1].

The term "skills" implies abilities that are predominantly based on learning experiences. Consequently, SST uses behavioral therapy principles and techniques for teaching individuals to communicate their emotions and requests so that they are more likely to achieve their goals and meet their needs for the affiliative relationships and roles required for independent living. Transformed into the SST venue, the use of discriminative stimuli encompasses the trainer's prompting, cueing, instructing, and coaching of individuals, where the latter involves practicing improved social behaviors. Because these instructional strategies increase the likelihood of more skillful social performance, they are associated with positive reinforcement contingent upon improved communication. Applications of social learning theory to the acquisition of instrumental skills include the use of modeling and other modes of observational learning. When individuals are reinforced by achieving interpersonal goals, their likelihood of initiating future social communications increases. Learning theory shows that observable behaviors are more accessible to therapeutic intervention and thus more readily acquired and modified than covert cognitions and emotions. Thoughts and feelings are subjectively experienced behavioral responses that constantly interact in a reciprocal manner with obvious behaviors such as verbal and nonverbal communications. Because social competence is strengthened through the successful use of social skills in community life, cognitions and emotions also shift in positive ways with improvements in self-efficacy, self-esteem, self-confidence, empowerment, optimism, and mood. Since the social skills used in everyday life can receive favorable responses from a person's social network, desired changes occur at the subjective level of experience. SST can be carried out by individuals, families, or groups, each with its own advantages [2]. The advantage of SST conducted individually is that the training process and skills can be acquired rapidly. On the other hand, the advantage of conducting SST with families or groups is the ability to make it readily generalizable to the home and everyday life. There are various modalities of SST, which are still in the developmental stage and expected to be improved in the future to acquire more social functions.

3 Participants

SST has been widely used for people with psychiatric disorders. Among these, the etiology of schizophrenia is thought to be largely related to social factors, and thus SST was first used for people with this psychiatric disorder [3, 4]. On the other hand, although it is believed that people with neurodevelopmental disorders have had the core symptoms since childhood, their mental symptoms are thought to worsen due to environmental factors, including social factors. Therefore, improving the social skills of individuals suffering from neurodevelopmental issues will lessen their core symptoms and prevent secondary psychiatric disorders [5]. SST is thus considered effective for people with schizophrenia and neurodevelopmental disorders, with various studies arguing the usefulness of SST [6, 7].

In this study's research, we conducted SST on adults with schizophrenia, those with ASD, and HC adults for a comparative perspective. Adults with schizophrenia and with ASD were assessed by two or more experienced psychiatrists using the Diagnostic and Statistical Manual of Mental Disorders, Fifth Edition (DSM-5). We gathered 49 adult subjects: 19 HC adults (10 males and 9 females; mean age 28.42 years, with standard deviation of 3.95 years), 16 with ASD (10 males, 6 females; age: $M = 26.50$, $SD = 5.67$), and 15 with schizophrenia (7 males, 8 females; age: $M = 32.07$, $SD = 8.82$). The data collection period was from January 2020 to January 2021.

We also studied 18 HC adults to assess the effects of automated SST. We randomly divided HC adults into two groups: 9 in the automated SST group and 9 in the control group (no SST), and we later compared them retrospectively. The data collection period was from July 2022 to August 2022.

We excluded participants with a history of psychiatric hospitalization from the HC group. We also excluded participants who scored less than 70 points on the Wechsler Adult Intelligence Scale-Third Edition (WAIS-III), an intelligence quotient test. In addition, we excluded participants with drug or alcohol addictions, personality disorders, or organic—including symptomatic—psychiatric disorders. The sample size was set to balance the generality of the results and the practical workload of data collection.

All participants provided written informed consent after receiving an explanation of the study procedures. This study was conducted in accordance with the Declaration of Helsinki of the World Medical Association and was approved by the ethics committees of Nara Institute of Science and Technology and Nara Medical University.

4 Assessment

Bellack outlined a number of strategies employed in the assessment of social skills. The most commonly employed of these assessments are self-reporting and self-monitoring, as well as behavioral observation. The evaluation scales used in SST are mainly those related to social skills, while the other scales are for evaluating the symptoms of the psychiatric disorder suffered by the participant. In this study, we also decided to use a scale for social anxiety, which affects communication, and a scale for self-efficacy, which affects participation in society.

The Kikuchi Social Skills Scale [8] (KiSS-18) in Japanese, the Social Responsiveness Scale 2nd edition [9] (SRS-2) (Japanese version [10]), and the Singelis Self-Construal Scale [11] (SCS) (Japanese version [12]) are self-assessment measures used to examine social functioning. KiSS-18 measures the level of social skills and consists of 18 questions based on six categories of social skills as defined by Kikuchi. SRS-2 measures the severity of social impairment and consists of 65 questions. SCS is a 7-point rating scale, for 30 questions, that measures independent self-construal and interdependent self-construal.

In the study evaluating the effects of automated SST and human–human SST for HC adults, we used the State-Trait Anxiety Inventory [13] (STAI) (Japanese version [14]) and Liebowitz Social Anxiety Scale [15] (LSAS) (Japanese version [16]) to examine social anxiety as self-assessment scales. The General Self-Efficacy Scale [17] (GSES) (Japanese version [18]) was used as a self-assessment scale to evaluate self-efficacy. STAI has 20 items for assessing trait anxiety and 20 for state anxiety rated on a 4-point scale. LSAS is designed to evaluate the range and severity of social anxiety disorder and has 24 items on a scale 0–3 to rate the level of fear and the degree to which the situation can be avoided. GSES is a 10-item psychometric scale designed to assess optimistic self-beliefs for coping with a variety of difficult demands in life.

Although self-assessment measures can provide valuable data, they have their limitations. For example, it would be difficult to self-monitor appropriate eye contact. In addition, there are problems with validity and reliability, especially the latter, which may change an individual's self-assessment criteria within a given period of time.

Therefore, we conducted two behavioral observational assessments: the Face Emotion Identification Test [19] (FEIT) and the second edition of the Autism Diagnostic Observation Schedule [20] (ADOS-2). For adults, FEIT assesses facial emotion recognition and consists of 21 face images with one of 7 emotions (happiness, sadness, fear, anger, surprise, disgust, and neutral) on a gray scale. FEIT scores were calculated as the number of correct answers for each task. We used Tobii Pro Fusion [21] to measure eye movement. ADOS-2 is a semi-structured assessment that includes several play-based activities to gather information on communication, social interaction, and limiting and repetitive behaviors associated with ASD.

An assessment of the behaviors related to interpersonal skills during the SST role-plays was also conducted. The role-play situations were set up to use Bellack's four fundamental social skills. We prepared four variations for each of these four fundamental social skills. Bellack's four fundamental social skills are explained in more detail in the following section on training. We used video cameras and Kinect to capture the SST role-play for evaluation. Two video cameras were placed behind each participant to record the other from an oblique angle. A wider video of both participants was also recorded, and two Kinect sensors were installed at the sides. Due to Covid-19 concerns, a transparent partition was placed between the participant and trainer (Fig. 1). Third-party psychiatrists watched the recorded video from the oblique and side views. We adopted a revised role-play test [22]. Two psychiatrists used a Likert scale from 1 to 5 to evaluate eye contact, body orientation and distance, facial expression, voice variation, clarity, fluency, and social appropriateness while watching the recorded video. The two psychiatrists who assessed the participants were blind to each participant's diagnosis and background.

In addition, only for the Schizophrenia group, we used the Japanese version of the Brief Assessment of Cognition in Schizophrenia [23] (BACS-J) to evaluate cognitive function and the Positive and Negative Syndrome Scale [24] (PANSS) to evaluate the severity of schizophrenia symptoms.

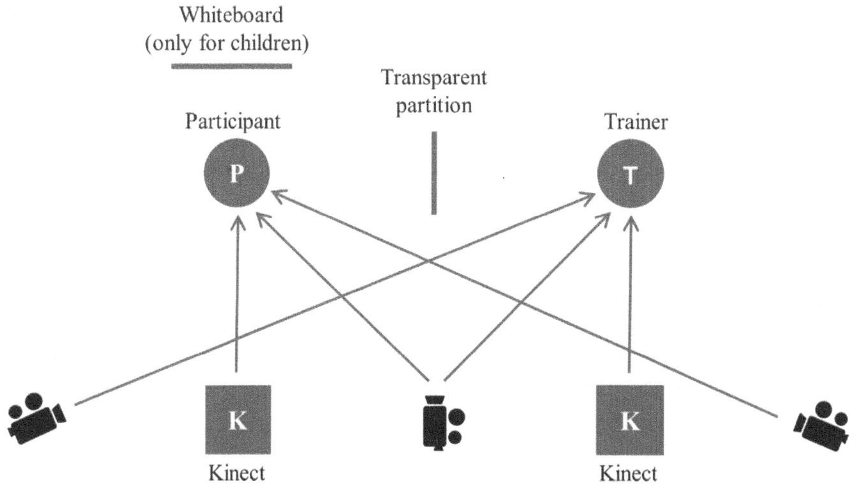

Fig. 1 SST recording setup

5 Training

R.P. Liberman presented a prototypical SST session [25]: As an introduction step, an explanation is given of why and how to conduct SST. After this introduction, the participant is asked to act out an interpersonal situation with a trainer or a fellow participant. Next, the trainer reviews the participant's performance and reinforces the correct behavior that would result in a more socially appropriate performance. This cycle is repeated until the performance meets the criteria specified by the trainer. Videotapes may be used to assist in the reviewing process. Modeling and coaching may be used to demonstrate and prompt more effective behaviors, but instructions alone are usually effective enough. The focus of feedback is almost always on the topography of the participant's performance. The two main types of behaviors are non-content behaviors, such as eye contact, speech disturbance, smiling, voice intonation, response duration, response latency, posture, and use of hand gestures, and, on the other hand, content-related behaviors, such as the frequency of behavior-change requests as well as expressions of compliance, independence, appreciation, affection, and hostility. Every SST, without exception, includes one or more of these behaviors in its training programs. This suggests a shared conceptual definition of social skills in terms of their topographical features. Acquiring adequate social skills is conceptualized as addressing an inadequate incidence of the topographical features that are the focus of attention in the feedback process, and it is presumed that increasing this incidence through instruction, modeling, coaching, and reinforcement will enhance social skills, which in turn will increase the potential for community adaptation. Homework is frequently used to extend the effectiveness of training beyond the immediate session. Homework assignments are tasks that require patients to practice, outside of the session, the behaviors they have been taught to gain greater social proficiency. Homework prompts "real-world" performances that directly lead to satisfying the participant's needs, desires, and interpersonal relationships. Homework may be used to extend the effectiveness of training beyond a specific session, but training time and the number of interpersonal situations that can be covered are limited [26]. Table 1 summarizes the common patterns of the prototypical SST according to Liberman.

Table 1 Common pattern of prototypical SST according to Liberman

1.	Evaluate participants' weaknesses and strengths in interpersonal situations
2.	Provide a way to learn specific social skills
3.	Model social skills in simulated social situations
4.	Given instructions that focus on certain social skills that the participant should practice
5.	Have participants role-play a certain social skill
6.	Provide participants with positive and corrective feedback
7.	Repeated Role-play and feedback
8.	Provide homework to encourage generalization

We arranged SST along the lines of the prototypical SST to compare human–human SST and automated SST. In prototypical SST, social skills in daily life are first assessed for each participant, social skills to be trained are selected, and the need for training in those social skills is explained. However, since it was difficult to adapt the social skills trained to each participant in automated SST, the four fundamental social skills proposed by A.S. Bellack were used [27]. These four fundamental social skills are listening, expressing positive or negative feelings, asking for favors, and declining requests (we call these "LISTEN," "TELL," "ASK," and "DECLINE" in the rest of this chapter). We explained the need for each of these four basic social skills before we trained them, and then we conducted SST. First, the social skill of "LISTEN" states, "During a conversation, it is important to show the other person that you are listening and paying attention to what they are saying the whole time. When the other person sees that you are listening, they will want to continue the conversation further. Now let's practice listening to what the other person has to say"; the trainer gave this explanation in Japanese and then began the role-play for the "LISTEN" skill. The social skill of "TELL" states, "When you express gratitude for what others have done for you, it strengthens your sense of belonging as a peer and that you can do well. Now let's practice expressing gratitude to others"; the trainer explained this and began the role-play of the "TELL" skill. The social skill of "ASK" states, "We all ask people to do something in our lives, or we ask them to change their behavior. If you tell them in a way that they don't feel uncomfortable, it is easier for them to comply with your request. Now let's train asking for a favor"; the trainer explained this and began the role-play of the "ASK" skill. Finally, the social skill of "DECLINE" states, "When people ask you to do something, you don't always do what they want. It is important to say no in a way that the other person doesn't feel bad. Let's practice saying no to a request"; the trainer explained this and began the role-play of the "DECLINE" skill.

Participants are assigned roles and demonstrate them according to the prepared scenario. After the role-play by the participants, the participants discuss their findings and impressions from this activity. The trainer also provides feedback to the participants on what was good and what could have been improved. Role-plays by participants may be repeated and redone. We created 4 role-play variations for each of the 4 tasks. The role-play variations included the following scenarios: in a hospital, at home, at school, at the workplace, and with friends. We used a visual radar chart for each assessment item in automated SST (eye contact, body direction and distance, facial expression, vocal variation, clarity, fluency, and social appropriateness) to provide feedback. In the human–human SST, the trainer referred to each of the assessment items also used in the automated SST and then provided feedback. Although the trainer provides feedback, we decided to have only one role-play by the participants, without any subsequent one.

It appears that SST is powerful in shaping new behaviors in the training, but there are problems with the generalization of these newly acquired social skills to the natural environment. Generalizing the social skills learned into daily life requires modifying the use of those skills on a case-by-case basis to suit the situation. For this reason, assigning homework is important in generalizing learned social skills in

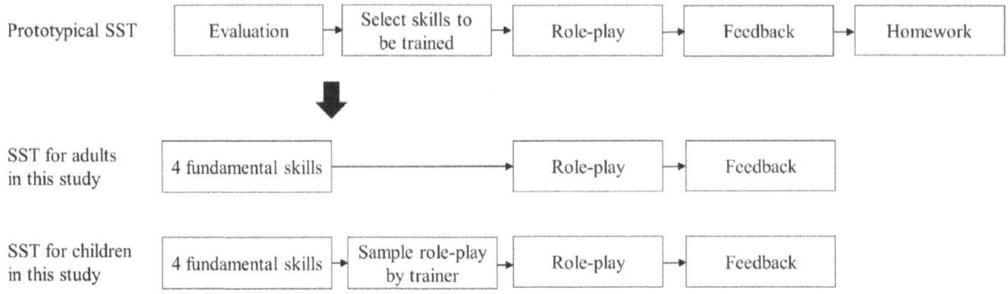

Fig. 2 Flowchart of each SST

daily life. In this study, however, homework was omitted due to the complexity of setting homework in automated SST as well as our research purpose of evaluating the effectiveness of automated SST. A flowchart of the SST is shown in Fig. 2.

We made comparisons among the assessments of adults with schizophrenia, adults with ASD, and HC adults. In addition, in other HC adults, to compare the effects of automated SST, the participants were randomly divided into an automated SST group and a control group. One week after the pre-evaluation, each SST was done four times over four weeks, followed by a post-evaluation one week later. Please see the following chapters for descriptions of participant demographics and rating scale results for the adult SST.

6 Social Skills Training (SST) for Children

Liberman's basic framework of SST developed in the 1970s was mainly for chronic psychiatric disorders such as schizophrenia, but SST for children has a longer history and has been used since the 1960s to train children whenever there are concerns about maladjustment [28]. Lack of social skills is common in children and adolescents with psychiatric disorders. SST is a component of behavioral therapy, the purpose of which is to "promote the acquisition of skills, to refine skills already acquired, and to enable the application of social skills to different situations and people." SST is often conducted in a group format that allows children and adolescents to practice their newly acquired skills with peers [29]. The intended social skills vary depending on the current concerns of the children and adolescents. For example, children/adolescents who internalize feelings need to be trained to talk to others about themselves and to initiate conversations on their own, while giving and receiving compliments. In contrast, children/adolescents who externalize their feelings require training in empathy. Training of these children and adolescents focuses on conflict resolution techniques, such as walking away from a situation, ignoring, and accepting or interacting with feelings. SST is often used in the treatment of children and adolescents, especially those with ASD, who, depending on their severity, require intensive training based on shaping. Shaping, introduced by Skinner, is a conditioning paradigm used primarily in the experimental analysis of behavior. The method used is differential reinforcement of successive approximations [30].

Children have more difficulty than adults in responding flexibly and understanding the context of conversations. Therefore, in SST for children, it is important to construct a standardized program, visualize what needs to be understood, and make the modeling easy to understand. Children also have difficulty in generalizing the skills they learn in SST to the real world. Therefore, it is effective for those adults who will be present in the child's naturalistic social interactions (e.g., parents and teachers) to engage in SST for children. In addition, there are SST programs that are peer-mediated and embedded in naturalistic settings. For example, in Children's Friendship Training (CFT), in which parents are involved in the treatment process for the first time to ensure generalization to school and home, parents' ratings of social skills were higher after training than in a group that did not involve parents in the treatment process, and these ratings were maintained even three months after training [31].

7 Participants

In neurodevelopmentally challenged individuals, early social cognitive intervention from childhood is strongly advocated. Accordingly, SST for children with neurodevelopmental disorders is effective in terms of developing social skills and preventing secondary psychiatric disorders [32]. On the other hand, schizophrenia is a psychiatric disorder that generally develops during adolescence and adulthood, so there are few children with schizophrenia.

Therefore, we conducted SST on children with ASD and TD children for a comparative study. Children with ASD were assessed by two or more experienced psychiatrists using the Diagnostic and Statistical Manual of Mental Disorders, Fifth Edition (DSM-5). We collected 33 child subjects ranging in age from 8 to 13 years old: 17 TD children (9 males and 8 females; mean age was 10.82 years, standard deviation of age was 1.55 years) and 16 children with ASD (13 males and 3 females; M = 11.0, SD = 1.37). We excluded participants with a history of psychiatric hospitalization from the TD children group. We excluded participants who scored less than 70 points on the Wechsler Intelligence Scale for Children-Fourth Edition (WISC-IV), an intelligence quotient test, from both groups. In addition, we excluded participants with psychiatric disorders other than ASD, defined by the DSM-5, a neurological disorder, a head injury, a serious medical condition, or a history of substance abuse or dependence. The sample size was set to balance the generality of the results and the practical workload of data collection. The data collection period was from April 2021 to July 2021.

All participants and their parents provided written informed consent after receiving an explanation on the study procedures. This study was conducted in accordance with the Declaration of Helsinki of the World Medical Association and was approved by the ethics committees of Nara Institute of Science and Technology and Nara Medical University.

8 Assessment

Children have more difficulty evaluating themselves objectively than adults, and it is especially difficult for children with ASD to evaluate themselves objectively. Therefore, in addition to the child's own subjective evaluation, the evaluation of parents, teachers, and others close to the child, as well as objective evaluations, are more important than for adults. Furthermore, the ASD group was not evaluated by the children themselves but rather by their parents and objective evaluations.

KIDSCREEN-10 [32] (Japanese version [33]) and the Rosenberg Self-Esteem Scale [34] (RSES-J, Japanese version [35]) were used as self-administered tests by the participant children themselves. KIDSCREEN-10 and RSES were assessed only for the TD Children. KIDSCREEN-10 is a 10-item test designed to examine overall health-related aspects of children's quality of life. RSES is a 10-item, 4-point Likert-type scale that measures children's self-esteem. In addition to the children's own ratings, SRS-2 [9, 10], ADHD Rating Scale IV [36] (ADHD-RS-IV) (Japanese version [37]), and the Strengths and Difficulties Questionnaire [38] (SDQ) (Japanese version [39]) were used as parental ratings. ADHD-RS-IV is a scale based on the DSM-IV, in which parents or teachers rate questions related to hyperactivity, impulsivity, and inattention, which are symptoms of attention-deficit/hyperactivity disorder (ADHD). SDQ is a 25-item questionnaire developed by Goodman to be answered by parents or teachers about children's emotions and behavior, and it is divided into subscales of emotional symptoms (ES), conduct problems (CP), hyperactivity/inattention (HI), peer problems (PP), and prosocial behavior (PB), and the total score of these subscales is calculated as the Total Difficulties Score (TDS). In addition, the problem scale of Child Behavior Checklist/4–18 [40] (CBCL/4–18) (Japanese version [41]) was conducted on the ASD children group. CBCL/4–18 was developed by Achenbach, and it consists of a Social Competence Scale and a Problem Scale. The Social Competence Scale is a questionnaire of the child's life situation, including favorite sports and hobbies, household chores the child does, and academic performance, while the Problem Scale is a questionnaire on emotional and behavioral problems, consisting of 118 questions and one writable item. The problem scale consists of 9 narrowband scales (aggressive behavior, anxious/depressed, attention problems, rule-breaking behavior, somatic complaints, social problems, thought problems, withdrawn/depressed, and other problems) and 2 broadband scales (internalizing problems and externalizing problems). The total problems score is the sum of all problem items' scores. The questionnaire is intended for ages 4–18, and it is to be completed by a parent or equivalent caregiver.

For the same reasons as in our adult study, we conducted objective assessment in children. As an objective assessment, we also conducted FEIT [42]. For children, FEIT assesses facial emotion recognition and consists of 32 face images with one of 4 emotions (happiness, sadness, anger, and surprise) on a gray scale. The FEIT scores were calculated as the number of correct answers for each task. We used Tobii Pro Fusion to measure eye movement.

As with the adults, we assessed interpersonal skills during SST role-plays in the SST for children. The role-play situations were also set up to use Bellack's four fundamental social skills. As with the SST for adults, the video cameras and Kinetic units were used to capture the SST role-play for evaluation. These devices were positioned in the same configuration, and the participant and trainer were filmed in the same way as in the SST for adults. Due to Covid-19 concerns, a transparent partition was placed between the participant and trainer (Fig. 1). One of the two third-party psychiatrists and two occupational therapists served as evaluators. The evaluators watched the recorded video from oblique and side views. We adopted a revised role-play test [21], where the evaluators used a Likert scale from 1 to 5 for eye contact, body orientation and distance, facial expression, voice variation, clarity, fluency, and social appropriateness while watching the recorded videos, in the same way as for the adults. The evaluators were blind to the participants' diagnoses and backgrounds.

9 Training

The SST program examined in this study is based on the Japanese version of the SST for children. This was originally designed and implemented by F. Frankel at the University of California, Los Angeles (UCLA) [43] and then revised by H. Iwasaka et al. [44]. In Iwasaka's SST version, since social skills are mainly used in play by children and intended to promote generalization in daily life, the program is divided into learning time for children to learn social skills, playing time for children to play using the learned social skills, and a parent program to show parents how they can help their children use the skills they have learned. The SST used in this study omitted playing time, due to time constraints, and thus focused on learning time so that parents could observe and learn from it. The SST in this study was not conducted with peers but with one child alone, since the automated SST was conducted in a one-on-one setting.

The SST program for children followed the same process as the SST for adults. However, since it was considered difficult for children to imagine the SST role-play situations, the trainers demonstrated a sample role-play before the role-play in which the children participated. Before the children conducted their role-play, the trainer and children simulated one-on-one how the role-play would be conducted.

In addition, to make it easier to understand what should be done in SST, we displayed posters to allow the children to visualize this. Basic communication skills such as "make eye contact," "use your hands to express yourself," "look forward to speaking," "look cheerful," "speak clearly," and "act appropriately for the story" were displayed on a whiteboard, and the trainers read the visualized social skills and told the participants to adhere to those skills. The skills learned in SST and why those skills are needed were also shown on the whiteboard, and the trainers read the visualization of the skills and the need for them each time before role-playing the use of those skills. The whiteboard was placed right next to the children when they were doing SST (Fig. 1). In addition, the position where the child stands during the role-play was indicated by tape on the floor.

The social skills set in this study's SST for children were the same four fundamental social skills of "LISTEN," "TELL," "ASK," and "DECLINE" as used in the SST for adults. Before the children role-played each of the four fundamental social skills, the trainers role-played a sample. First, the trainer asked why the participants needed the social skills they were about to learn and interacted with them. After that, the trainer read from a whiteboard a description of each skill to be learned and the need for that skill. Finally, the trainer performed a sample role-play using the given skill. The trainer explained that the "LISTEN" skill is the skill of listening to others, and that it is necessary because "replying and responding to others makes them feel good" and "lets you know what the people with whom you talk are thinking." In the case of the "TELL" skill, the trainer explained that it is the skill of communicating your feelings and that it is necessary to "make people understand what you are thinking." In the "ASK" skill, the trainer explained that it is the skill of making a valid request and that it is necessary for "getting people to understand what you want them to do" and "getting them to help you with something you can't do yourself." Finally, the trainer explained that the skill of "DECLINE" is the skill of being able to say no effectively and that it is necessary to "make people understand that you can't do something" and to "avoid making them feel bad."

Participants are assigned roles and demonstrated them according to the prepared scenario. The scenarios were simpler than those for adults, and for children who were anxious about role-playing, the trainer explained in advance what to say and when to say it by showing them the lines on paper or by discussing the situation in detail with the child before the role-play. Since the role-play variations were intended for children, the situations were mainly set up at home, at school, or among friends. For each of the four skills, about three variations were prepared, and the variations were tailored to the children's interests. For example, in role-play using the "LISTEN" skill, the trainer talks about the children's hobby. In the role-play using the "TELL" skill, the trainer might set up a situation in which the children thank their mothers for their hospitality. In the role-play using the "ASK" skill, the trainer might create a situation in which the children ask their friends to play outside. In the role-play using the "DECLINE" skill, the trainer might set up a situation in which they decline their mothers' request to help because they have something to do.

Finally, the trainers gave the children feedback on their role-plays. In those feedback sessions, the trainer gave positive feedback on what was done and what could be done even better in the role-play. The SST for children provided a greater proportion of positive feedback than the SST conducted for adults to motivate their learning of social skills. Only one role-play was carried out by the participants for each skill. In the SST for children in this study, homework was omitted, as in the SST for adults. A flowchart of this study's SST for children is shown in Fig. 2.

In this study, we assessed and compared TD children and children with ASD. FEIT could not be performed in only 1 of the 16 participants in the ASD group. Table 2 gives detailed data, including rating scales for the ASD and TD groups, and Table 3 gives the scales of the revised role-play test for these groups.

Table 2 Participants' characteristics

	TD (n = 17)	ASD (n = 16)	
Sex	M: 9 F: 8	M: 13 F: 3	
Assessment	Average(SD)	Average(SD)	p value
Age	10.82(1.55)	11.00(1.37)	0.732
KIDSCREEN-10	44.29(4.36)	N.A	N.A
RSES	29.65(5.45)	N.A	N.A
SRS-2	22.41(14.15)	74.69(25.96)	<0.001**
ADHD-RS-IV	6.88(9.40)	17.13(10.05)	0.005**
SDQ: Emotional symptoms	0.88(1.05)	2.63(2.19)	0.009**
SDQ: Conduct problems	1.06(1.48)	2.25(1.73)	0.041*
SDQ: Hyperactivity/inattention	2.35(2.37)	5.25(2.54)	0.002**
SDQ: Peer problems	0.94(1.68)	4.06(2.52)	<0.001**
SDQ: Prosocial behavior	7.94(2.25)	3.50(2.25)	<0.001**
SDQ: Total difficulty score	5.24(5.33)	14.19(4.92)	<0.001**
CBCL: Total problems score	N.A	37.19(14.09)	N.A
CBCL: Internalizing problems	N.A	9.75(6.23)	N.A
CBCL: Externalizing problems	N.A	8.81(7.82)	N.A
CBCL: Aggressive behavior	N.A	7.38(6.34)	N.A
CBCL: Anxious/depressed	N.A	5.56(3.79)	N.A
CBCL: Attention problems	N.A	7.69(3.28)	N.A
CBCL: Rule-Breaking Behavior	N.A	1.44(1.79)	N.A
CBCL: Somatic Complaints	N.A	0.94(2.24)	N.A
CBCL: Social Problems	N.A	5.81(2.59)	N.A
CBCL: Thought Problems	N.A	1.31(1.30)	N.A
CBCL: Withdrawn/Depressed	N.A	3.38(2.47)	N.A
CBCL: Other Problems	N.A	5.81(4.18)	N.A
FEIT	22.18(2.72)	20.67(3.72)	0.196

Table 3 Participants' characteristics of revised role-play test

		TD (n = 17)	ASD (n = 16)	
Social Skill	Assessment Item	Average(SD)	Average(SD)	p Value
Listen	eye contact	4.61(0.60)	3.53(0.87)	<0.001**
	body orientation and distance	4.09(0.57)	3.13(1.04)	0.003**
	facial expression	4.38(0.65)	2.47(0.78)	<0.001**
	voice variation	4.27(0.73)	2.59(0.74)	<0.001**
	clarity	4.62(0.45)	3.09(0.55)	<0.001**
	fluency	4.56(0.50)	3.03(0.74)	<0.001**
	social appropriateness	4.59(0.40)	2.81(0.73)	<0.001**
Tell	eye contact	4.56(0.58)	3.50(0.98)	<0.001**
	body orientation and distance	4.35(0.58)	3.19(0.96)	<0.001**
	facial expression	4.38(0.57)	2.93(0.95)	<0.001**
	voice variation	4.27(0.66)	2.88(0.99)	<0.001**
	clarity	4.65(0.46)	3.19(0.96)	<0.001**
	fluency	4.47(0.60)	2.91(1.02)	<0.001**
	social appropriateness	4.56(0.56)	3.06(0.83)	<0.001**
Ask	eye contact	4.53(0.65)	3.72(0.63)	0.001**
	body orientation and distance	4.27(0.79)	3.28(1.00)	0.004**
	facial expression	4.41(0.59)	2.90(0.78)	<0.001**
	voice variation	4.47(0.41)	2.81(0.73)	<0.001**
	clarity	4.79(0.40)	3.25(0.71)	<0.001**
	fluency	4.56(0.43)	3.03(0.78)	<0.001**
	social appropriateness	4.35(0.61)	3.12(0.50)	<0.001**
Decline	eye contact	4.47(0.62)	3.66(0.65)	<0.001**
	body orientation and distance	4.14(0.86)	3.12(0.85)	0.002**
	facial expression	4.21(0.69)	2.56(0.70)	<0.001**
	voice variation	4.32(0.64)	2.66(0.79)	<0.001**
	clarity	4.71(0.69)	3.41(0.80)	<0.001**
	fluency	4.59(0.48)	2.84(0.63)	<0.001**
	social appropriateness	4.35(0.72)	3.03(0.74)	<0.001**

Group differences tested with t-test
** $P < 0.01$

10 The Need for Automated SST-Based Technology

SST is one of the most commonly used interventions for helping people who lack interpersonal skills to learn those skills at all ages, from children to adults, and it is also useful for patients with chronic psychiatric disorders. Human–human SST is the traditional type, and although it is effective as an intervention to learn interpersonal skills, there are barriers to using it to conduct SST. Specifically, human–human SST requires multiple facilitators who are SST experts, as well as the time and the place for training or the need to travel distances. This makes accessibility to SST difficult, especially for those who are economically distressed or unable to find the time for SST. There was also the Covid-19 pandemic, which made accessibility to SST even more difficult. In addition, facilitators have to make the time for SST while also devoting time to their regular duties, and SST is not cost-effective because it requires time and several facilitators. Moreover, the effectiveness of SST varies with the conditions and skill of the facilitators.

In recent years, technology-based SSTs have been developed to make this treatment available at convenient times and at low cost [45]. Some possible advantages of technology-based SST include the ability to reduce anxiety about interpersonal situations, to set up an environment that facilitates concentration, and to visualize feedback. Furthermore, as Artificial Intelligence (AI) and Virtual Reality (VR) technologies develop, it will be possible to flexibly learn more varied social skills in different virtual situations. Some technology-based SSTs use computer software [46], some use human-like avatars [47], and some use therapeutic robots [48]. In addition, these technology-based SSTs have been reported to improve social skills [45]. Therefore, it is expected that technology-based SSTs will expand the options for using SST.

Of course, it is important to engage with people in the real world to truly learn interpersonal skills. Human–human SSTs have advantages over technology-based SSTs in that trainers and participants can develop relationships and expand those relationships to others. With this understanding, it will continue to be necessary to find effective ways to make the best use of automated SSTs.

References

1. T. Amagasa, Social Skills Training: How to use it and practice more effective? Japanese Journal of Clin Psychiatr. **63**(10), 1483–1490 (2021)
2. A. Kopelowicz, R.P. Liberman, R. Zarate, Recent advances in social skills training for schizophrenia. Schizophr Bull. **32**(Suppl 1), S12–23 (2006)
3. S.L. Kerr, J.M. Neale, Emotion perception in schizophrenia: specific deficit or further evidence of generalized poor performance? T Adnorm Psychol **102**(2), 312–318 (1993)
4. A.S. Bellack, K.T. Mueser, S. Gingerich, J. Agresta. *Social Skills Training for Schizophrenia: A Step-by Step Guide.* 2nd ed. (Guilford Press, 2004)
5. C.T. Moody, E.A. Laugeson, Social Skills Training in Autism Spectrum Disorder Across the Lifespan. Child Adolesc. Psychiatr. Clin. N. Am. **29**(2), 359–371 (2020)
6. M. Solmi, G. Croatto, G. Piva, S. Rosson, P. Fusar-Poli, J.M. Rubio, A.F. Carvalho, E. Vieta, C. Arango, N.R. Detore, E.S. Eberlin, K.T. Mueser, C.U. Correll, Efficacy and acceptability of psychosocial interventions in schizophrenia: systematic overview and quality appraisal of the meta-analytic evidence. Mol. Psychiatry **28**(1), 354–368 (2023)
7. J. Dubreucq, F. Haesebaert, J. Plasse, M. Dubreucq, N. Franck, A Systematic Review and Meta-analysis of Social Skills Training for Adults with Autism Spectrum Disorder. J. Autism Dev. Disord. **52**(4), 1598–1609 (2022)

8. A. Kikuchi, The social skills are measured. Article in Japanese in *Shakaiteki Skill o Hakaru: KiSS-18 Handbook*, (Kawashima Shoten, Tokyo, 2007), pp. 1–204
9. J.N. Constantino, C.P. Gruber, Social responsiveness scale: SRS-2. Western psychological services, (2012)
10. Y. Kamio, N. Inada, A. Moriwaki, M. Kuroda, T. Koyama, H. Tsujii, Y. Kawakubo, H. Kuwabara, K.J. Tsuchiya, Y. Uno, J.N. Constantino, Quantitative autistic traits ascertained in a national survey of 22529 Japanese schoolchildren. Acta Psychiatr. Scand. **128**(1), 45–53 (2013)
11. T.M. Singelis, The measurement of independent and interdependent self-construals. Pers. Soc. Psychol. Bull. **20**(5), 580–591 (1994)
12. T. Takata, M. Omoto, M. Seike, Construction of a revised scale for independent and interdependent construal of self. Memoir of the Nara University. **24**, 157–173 (1995)
13. C.D. Spielberger, State-trait anxiety inventory for adults. APA PsycTest. (1983)
14. N. Hidano, M. Fukuhara, M. Iwawaki, S. Soga, C.D. Spielberger, State trait anxiety inventory (form jyz). Article in Japanese. Japan UNI Agency. Tokyo, (2000)
15. M.R. Liebowitz, Social phobia. Mod. Probl. Pharmacopsychiatry **22**, 141–171 (1987)
16. S. Asakura, S. Inoue, F. Sasaki, Y. Sasaki, N. Kitagawa, T. Inoue, K. Denda, M. Ito, R. Matsubara, T. Koyama, Liebowitz social anxiety scale—Japanese version. APA PsycTest. (2002)
17. R. Schwarzer, M. Jerusalem, General seif-efficacy scale. APA PsycTest. (1995)
18. K. Narita, Y. Shimonaka, K. Nakazato, C. Kawaai, S. Sato, Y. Osada, A Japanese version of the generalized self-efficacy scale. Japanese J Educ Psychol. **43**(3), 306–314 (1995)
19. Facial emotion identification test for adult. 2020. Accessed on 05 May 2021
20. C. Lord, M. Rutter *Autism Diagnostic Observation Schedule,* 2nd ed. (WPS, 2012)
21. Tobii Pro Fusion. *Tobii Pro Fusion User's Manual.* (Tobii Pro, Danderyd, Sweden, 2019)
22. T. Sasaki, The reliability and validity of the revised role play test for assessment of social skills in schizophrenia. Clinical Psychiatry. **48**(11), 1191–1198 (2006)
23. R.S. Keefe, T.E. Goldberg, P.D. Harvey, J.M. Poe, L. Coughenour, The brief assessment of cognition in schizophrenia: reliability, sensitivity, and comparison with a standard neurocognitive battery. Schizophr. Res. **68**(2–3), 283–297 (2004)
24. S.R. Kay, A. Fiszbein, L.A. Opler, The positive and negative syndrome scale (PANSS) for schizophrenia. Schizophr. Bull. **13**(2), 261–276 (1987)
25. R.P. Liberman, *Personal effectiveness: Guiding People to Assert Themselves and Improve Their Social Skills.* (Research Press, 1975), pp.1–169
26. J. Prasko, I. Krone, J. Burkauskas, J. Vanek, M. Abeltina, A. Juskiene, T. Sollar, I. Bite, M. Slepecky, M. Ocikova, Homework in cognitive behavioral supervision: theoretical background and clinical application. Psychol. Res. Behav. Manag. **15**, 3809–3824 (2022)
27. A.S. Bellack, T. Kim, Mueser, S. Gingerich, J. Agresta, *Social Skills Training for Schizophrenia: A Step-by Step Guide*, 2nd ed. (Guilford Press, 2004)
28. S. Bellini, J. Peter, Social skills training for youth with autism spectrum disorders. Child Adolesc. Psychiatr. Clin. N. Am. **17**(4), 857–873 (2008)
29. G.B. Peterson, A day of great illumination: B.F. Skinner's discovery of shaping. J Exp Anal Behav. **82**(3), 317–28 (2004)
30. F. Frankel, R. Myatt, C. Sugar, C. Whitham, C.M. Gorospe, E. Langeson, A randomized controlled study of parent-assisted children's friendship training with children having autism spectrum disorders. J. Autism Dev. Disord. **40**(7), 827–842 (2010)
31. O.N. Choque, O. Flygare, C. Coco, A. Görling, A. Råde, Q. Chen, K. Lindstedt, S. Berggren, E. Serlachius, U. Jonsson, K. Tammimies, L. Kjellin, S. Bölte, Social skills training for children and adolescents with autism spectrum disorder: a randomized controlled trial. J. Am. Acad. Child Adolesc. Psychiatry **56**(7), 585–592 (2017)
32. U. Ravens-Sieberer, P. Auquier, M. Erhart, A. Gosch, L. Rajmil, J. Bruil, M. Power, W. Duer, B. Cloetta, L. Czemy, J. Mazur, A. Czimbalmos, Y. Tountas, C. Hagquist, J. Kilroe, European KIDSCREEN group. The KIDSCREEN-27 quality of life measure for children and adolescents: psychometric results from a cross-cultural survey in 13 European countries. Qual. Life Res. **16**, 1347–56 (2007)

33. S. Nezu, H. Iwasaka, K. Saeki, K. Obayashi, R. Ishizuka, H. Goma, Y. Furuichi, N. Kurumatani, Reliability and validity of Japanese version of KIDSCREEN-27 and KIDSCREEN-10 questionnaires. Environ. Health Prev. Med. **21**(3), 154–163 (2016)
34. M. Rosenberg, *Society and adolescent self-image* (Princeton University Press, New Jersey, 1965)
35. C. Mimura, P. Griffiths, A Japanese version of the Rosenberg self-esteem scale: translation and equivalence assessment. J Psychosomatic Res **62**, 589–594 (2007)
36. S. Zhang, D.E. Faries, M. Vowles, D. Michelson, ADHD rating scale IV: psychometric properties from a multinational study as a clinician-administered instrument. Int. J. Methods Psychiatr. Res. **14**(4), 186–201 (2005)
37. H. Ichikawa, K. Saito, T. Saito, N. Kariya, M. Kodaira, H. Ota, I. Kishida, K. Mikami, T. Ota, M. Kyo, H. Kosaka, F. Horiuchi, D. Okutsu, M. Fujiwara, A. Iwanami, Reliability and validity of the ADHD-RS-IV with adult prompts: the Japanese version. Japanese J Clin Psychiatr. **60**(4), 399–409 (2018)
38. R. Goodman, The strength and difficulties questionnaire: a research note. Japanese Child Psychol Psychiatry. **38**, 581–586 (1997)
39. W. Noda, H. Ito, S. Harada, Examining the reliability and validity of the Japanese version of the strengths and difficulties questionnaire self ratings form using the entire cohort data in one suburban city in Japan. Japanese J Clin Psychair **42**(1), 119–127 (2013)
40. T.M. Achenbach, C. Edelbrock, Child behavior checklist. Burlington (Vt). **7**, 371–392 (1991)
41. T. Itani, Y. Kanbayashi, Y. Nakata, M. Kita, H. Fujii, H. Kuramoto, Standardization of the Japanese version of the child behavior checklist/4-18. Psychiatria et Neurologia Paediatrica Japonica. **41**(4), 243–252 (2001)
42. Facial emotion identification test for child. 2020. Accessed on 14 May 2021
43. F. Frankel, R. Myatt, D.P. Cantwell, D.T. Feinberg, Parent-assisted transfer of children's social skills training: effect on children with and without attention-deficit hyperactivity disorder. J. Am. Acad. Child Adolesc. Psychiatry **36**(8), 1056–1064 (1997)
44. H. Iwasaka, H. Takahashi, Social skills training for ADHD. Jpn. J. Psychiatr. Treat. **25**(7), 911–918 (2010)
45. E.E. Soares, K. Bausback, C.L. Beard, M. Higinbotham, E.L. Bunge, G.W. Gengoux, Social skills training for autism spectrum disorders: a meta-analysis of in-person and technological interventions. J. Technol. Behav. Sci. **6**(1), 166–180 (2021)
46. M.L. Thomeer, R.A. Smith, C. Lopata, M.A. Volker, A.M. Lipinski, J.D. Rodger, C.A. McDonald, G.K. Lee, Randomized controlled trial of mind reading and in vivo rehearsal for high-functioning children with ASD. J. Autism Dev. Disord. **45**(7), 2115–2127 (2015)
47. L.M. Rice, C.A. Wall, A. Fogel, F. Shic, Computer-assisted face processing instruction improves emotion recognition, mentalizing, and social skills in students with ASD. J. Autism Dev. Disord. **45**(7), 2176–2186 (2015)
48. S. Yun, J. Choi, S. Park, G. Bong, H. Yoo, Social skills training for children with autism spectrum disorder using a robotic behavioral intervention system. Autism Res. **10**(7), 1306–1323 (2017)

Theory of Cognitive Behavioral Therapy

Takashi Kudo

1 Introduction

Cognitive Behavioral Therapy (CBT) is now being applied not only to depression and anxiety disorders but also to a wide range of psychiatric disorders. In Japan, in 2010, cognitive therapy and cognitive behavioral therapy, which are implemented by skilled physicians based on manuals for mood disorders, became eligible for medical reimbursement. Furthermore, in 2016, the scope was expanded to include anxiety disorders such as obsessive–compulsive disorder, social anxiety disorder, panic disorder, and post-traumatic stress disorder. In the United States, psychotherapy became mandatory during resident training in 2001, and subsequent revisions identified three specific types of psychotherapy: supportive psychotherapy, psychodynamic psychotherapy, and cognitive behavioral therapy. Today, CBT is not just a therapeutic approach one should be familiar with; it has become a practice that requires the ability to implement or appropriately refer alongside pharmacotherapy.

However, there are still misconceptions, such as the oversimplified notion that "CBT is a treatment method that uses activity logs or the column method." Such misunderstandings can lead to the improper application of CBT, which not only negatively impacts patients but also risks fostering further misunderstandings about the therapy itself.

In this review, I will outline the basic components of CBT, focusing on how it is based on specific models, how patients are understood through these models, and how this understanding is used within a framework to help improve the patient's issues. I will also examine the underlying neural mechanisms that form the basis of CBT.

T. Kudo (✉)
Osaka University, Osaka, Japan
e-mail: kudo@psy.med.osaka-u.ac.jp

S. Nakamura (ed.), *Multimodal Interaction Technologies for Training Affective Social Skills*, https://doi.org/10.1007/978-981-96-1313-7_4

2 Establishment of Cognitive Behavioral Therapy

Cognitive Behavioral Therapy (CBT) was established by Aaron Beck in the United States. The historical development of this approach is outlined below.

In 1959, Beck became an assistant professor of psychiatry at the University of Pennsylvania and began a study on dreams using depressed patients as part of his research to support psychoanalytic hypotheses. The specific psychoanalytic hypothesis he aimed to test was that "depression is caused by the inversion of hostility (aggression directed toward oneself)." However, contrary to this hypothesis, his experimental results led to the conclusion that "depressed individuals are not seeking failure; rather, they distort reality due to a negative view of themselves and their ability to achieve happiness." In other words, rather than interpreting dreams as a reflection of hidden (repressed) ideas or desires, it seemed more natural to view them as incorporating the patient's self-perception directly. This conclusion marked Beck's departure from psychoanalysis and paved the way for the establishment of his new theory of Cognitive Behavioral Therapy [1].

Around the same time, Beck made another important discovery: "automatic thoughts." While conducting free association with a depressed patient, the patient became angry and began to criticize Beck. When Beck inquired about the patient's feelings, the patient expressed surprising self-reproach, saying, "I shouldn't have said that. Blaming the doctor is wrong. He's going to dislike me." Beck found that other patients also harbored unspoken thoughts during therapy sessions. He termed these unspoken, involuntary thoughts "automatic thoughts." Beck realized that while these thoughts were not consciously recognized like voluntary thoughts, they annotated the patient's experiences. Furthermore, he found that in depressed individuals, these "automatic thoughts" were biased toward negativity [2].

In the 1970s, the field of psychology experienced a "cognitive revolution." This shift marked a transition from the operant model of behavioral therapy to a model that recognized and emphasized the role of information processing, i.e., cognition, in shaping human behavior and behavior change. This "cognitive revolution" influenced Beck and helped solidify the importance of cognition in CBT, distinguishing it from traditional behavioral therapies [3].

In 1979, Beck published Cognitive Therapy of Depression, based on his research up to that point, laying the foundation for CBT as it is practiced today.

3 Cognitive Behavioral Model

Taking action in response to environmental changes or stimuli is the essence of being a living organism. As organisms evolved, their sensory organs became more complex, and their capacity for memory increased. This necessitated the development of information processing systems that could gather, integrate, and process this

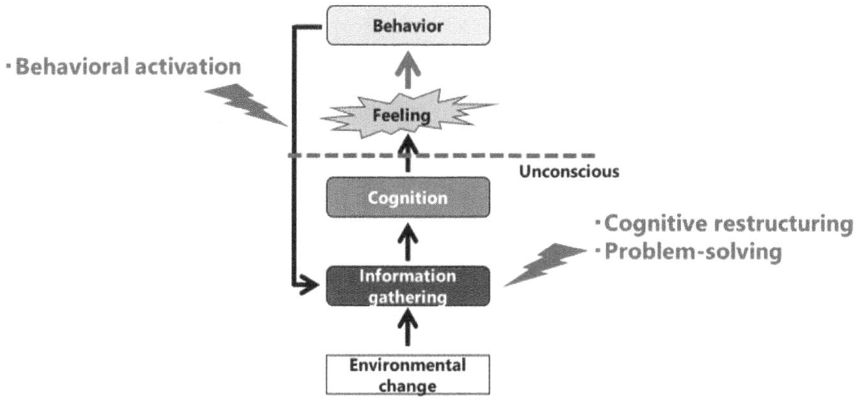

Fig. 1 Cognitive behavioral model

information in the brain to determine how to act. According to the "cognitive revolution," this information processing is synonymous with cognition. Moreover, in order to efficiently initiate behavior, a simplified cognitive process mediated by emotions evolved. In other words, this system developed to allow information processing to occur unconsciously, with behavior being driven by emotional responses as the monitor (Fig. 1).

The need for such simplified cognition can be attributed to the necessity of responding quickly in emergencies. For example, when encountering a predator, deciding how to respond and act is a matter of life or death. Cognition needs to happen instantaneously (without conscious awareness), emotions must be aroused, and behavior must follow immediately. This system allows for a rapid decision to either attack the opponent, driven by "anger," or flee from the threat, driven by "fear."

This system of cognition, based on simplification, is not only used in emergencies but is also widely employed in everyday life. However, if the information that forms the basis of cognition is accurate, there is no issue. But if the information is incorrect or insufficient, this rapid cognitive process—and the emotions that follow—will be flawed, leading to inappropriate actions. This forms the basis for the "cognitive behavioral model," which proposes that a patient's actions, emotions, or mood are largely influenced by their cognition.

The various tools of CBT focus on how to optimize the information gathered for this rapid cognitive process. Cognitive restructuring and problem-solving techniques aim to correct inaccurate or incomplete information, while behavioral activation can be interpreted as increasing the amount of information by prompting new experiences or utilizing past successes (memories) to expand the information base (Fig. 1).

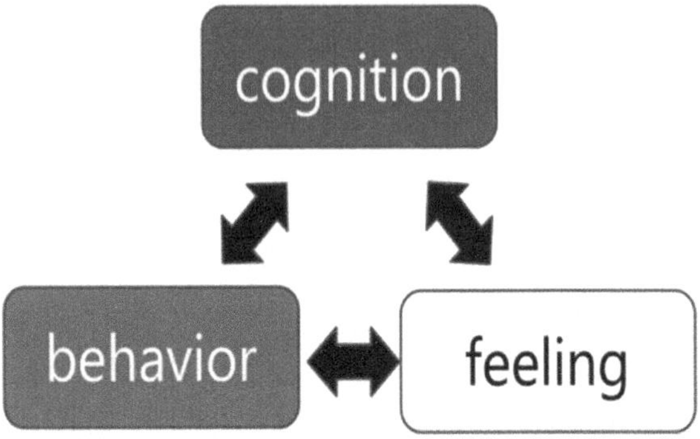

Fig. 2 Basic concepts of cognitive behavioral therapy

4 Basic Concepts of Cognitive Behavioral Therapy

Cognitive Behavioral Therapy (CBT) is based on the cognitive behavioral model, which suggests that a patient's mood and behavior are influenced by their cognition—how they perceive and interpret events (Fig. 2). Specifically, when a person encounters an event, pessimistic or negative cognitions about the event can lead to unpleasant moods and unhealthy behavioral patterns, creating a vicious cycle. While it is often difficult for patients to directly improve their mood, it is relatively easier to address and modify their cognitions and behaviors. By helping patients acquire adaptive thoughts and healthier behavioral patterns, CBT aims to improve their mood and break the negative cycle (Fig. 2).

In terms of the structure of cognition, it is believed that there are "automatic thoughts," which are spontaneous ideas or images that arise in response to a situation, and beneath these are deeper "schemas," which are shaped by the individual's worldview and values.

5 Collaborative Empiricism

In Cognitive Behavioral Therapy (CBT), the fundamental approach is a problem-solving one, where the therapist and patient work together to find solutions to problems occurring in the "here and now." While the term "problem-solving" might conjure a somewhat cold or clinical image, which can lead to misunderstandings about CBT, a strong therapeutic relationship is essential for collaborative problem-solving. Building this relationship requires basic therapeutic qualities that are foundational to all psychotherapies: empathy, warmth, and genuineness. These are fundamental in fostering collaboration as the therapist and patient work together to organize problems and explore solutions. This approach is referred to as "collaborative empiricism."

Throughout the sessions, various methods for solving problems are explored together, and it is crucial that the patient experiences these solutions in their daily life. While CBT is often called a self-care treatment, the aim is for the patient to gradually become their own therapist. Initially, the therapist takes the lead in guiding the process, but as therapy progresses, the patient assumes more responsibility until they are able to manage problem-solving independently.

As mentioned earlier, patients learn to handle their challenges through experience. Another key element in CBT is facilitating patient insight, and this is achieved using Socratic questioning, also known as guided discovery. Although CBT is considered an educational approach, it does not involve simply instructing the patient like a teacher would a student. For example, when reviewing an activity log (introduced later) with the patient, it would not be productive for the therapist to say, "It seems you have a tendency to do X." Instead, the therapist might ask, "Do you notice anything when you look at this log?" By asking questions in this way, the therapist helps the patient arrive at their own insights.

6 Structuring Therapy

Cognitive Behavioral Therapy (CBT) is known as a short-term, structured psychotherapy. This structure is designed to efficiently facilitate problem-solving and enhance the learning effect. Typically, CBT consists of 5 to 20 weekly sessions, each lasting 50 min. Depending on the disorder being treated, the duration of each session may be shortened, but regardless, the goal is to organize and narrow down the patient's problems within a limited timeframe and work toward resolving them.

The overall structure of CBT can be broadly divided into three phases: the early phase, the middle phase, and the final phase. In the early phase, an intake interview is conducted to gather information about the course of the patient's problems and to establish the therapeutic relationship. As the problems are further organized, a multi-faceted assessment is made to understand why the current condition has occurred and why it persists. This process leads to the conceptualization of the case and the setting of treatment goals. In the middle phase, the patient works on gaining skills tailored to the treatment plan that was established based on the treatment goals. In the final phase, the therapy is reviewed, and the therapist and patient discuss the skills acquired and measures for the future, with a focus on preventing relapse. It is also important to address any anxiety related to the termination of therapy. Furthermore, booster sessions may be scheduled to check whether the initial problems have resurfaced and whether the skills learned are being applied. If the issues have not been fully resolved, and it is determined that a few additional sessions could be effective, extending the number of sessions is also an option.

In addition to the overall structure, each session is also structured. Each session is divided into three main parts: the early part, the middle part, and the final part. At the beginning of the session, patients complete a questionnaire tailored to their disorder to check their symptoms. If there is a significant increase in suicidal ideation or feelings of hopelessness, a risk assessment is conducted, and it is considered whether these concerns should be added to the day's agenda. Since the goal here is to get an overview of the symptoms since the previous session, if the patient begins to talk in detail, the therapist might ask, "I'm sorry to interrupt, but could you briefly tell me how your depression or anxiety has been compared to last week?" Next, the agenda for the session is set. To make the most of the limited time and maximize effectiveness, only one or two agenda items are typically addressed per session. In the early stages, the therapist often leads the process of setting the agenda, but in later stages, patients usually take the lead. After the agenda is set, the therapist reviews what was discussed in the previous session to connect it to the current session. Lastly, the homework from the previous session is reviewed. Homework in CBT is not like schoolwork, where the teacher unilaterally assigns tasks to the student. Instead, it is an opportunity for the patient to practice the skills or concepts discussed in the session in their daily life. It is decided collaboratively during the session, and explaining to the patient that "homework is necessary to maximize the therapeutic effect by using what you've learned here in your everyday life" often helps reduce resistance and increases their motivation for treatment. Failing to review homework can negatively affect the therapeutic relationship and, in turn, the therapy itself, so it must be reviewed thoroughly. If the patient did not complete the homework, it should be considered whether this issue should be added to the session's agenda.

In the middle part of the session, the agenda is addressed, and any challenges or skills practiced are set as homework for the next session. During this time, the therapist provides feedback to ensure the patient's understanding of the content discussed. In the final part of the session, a review of the day's session is conducted. To ensure understanding, the patient is asked to summarize what was discussed. Additionally, the homework for the next session is confirmed, and the patient is asked to provide feedback to the therapist. Initially, many patients are hesitant to give feedback to their therapist, but explaining beforehand that "if the session progresses while you still have doubts, the therapeutic effect may not be as expected. Please feel free to speak up if you have any concerns so that we can work together on improving your symptoms and solving your problems" can positively contribute to building a strong therapeutic relationship and help the therapy proceed smoothly.

7 Case Conceptualization

Cognitive Behavioral Therapy (CBT) is not a treatment that simply applies techniques like cognitive restructuring or activity enhancement to patients. Whether for depression or anxiety disorders, the problems patients face vary greatly depending on their individual circumstances, making it essential to tailor CBT to each patient—essentially creating a customized approach. The comprehensive assessment of a patient's problems from past to present, and the framework for problem-solving, is known as case conceptualization (or formulation). Based on the following elements:

(1) diagnosis/symptoms, (2) formative influences, (3) situational issues, (4) biological, genetic, and medical factors, (5) strengths, (6) patterns of automatic thoughts, emotions, and behaviors, and (7) schemas, a working hypothesis is developed. Together with the patient, treatment goals are formulated, and a treatment plan to achieve those goals is implemented. Below are the key points for each of these elements.

For diagnosis/symptoms, the current symptoms are recorded in accordance with the diagnostic criteria of the DSM-5 (Diagnostic and Statistical Manual of Mental Disorders, 5th Edition). However, rather than merely noting the presence of symptoms, it is important to listen attentively to how these symptoms impact the patient's social and daily life. In formative influences, the therapist listens for events during the patient's developmental stages, the family history of mental illness, and family relationships, and how these factors may be contributing to current symptoms and interpersonal relationships. For situational issues, the therapist evaluates the triggering factors at the onset of the condition and the factors that sustain the symptoms, keeping both perspectives in mind. Multiple factors are often involved in the onset, and when evaluating sustaining factors, attention is also given to how the patient is responding to them. Biological, genetic, and medical factors should be recorded for both the patient and their family if applicable. In the strengths section, rather than focusing solely on negative aspects, attention is given to the patient's innate strengths and the strategies they have developed to cope despite their difficulties.

In terms of patterns of automatic thoughts, emotions, and behaviors, the therapist asks about three recent situations where the patient was distressed. Questions such as, "What thoughts or images came to mind when that event happened?" "How did you feel at that time?" and "What actions did you take?" are used to gather information and write down these patterns. For schemas, the therapist documents the schemas that were shaped by the patient's developmental history and past experiences. These schemas are revisited and refined as therapy progresses, becoming more accurate over time.

The working hypothesis is a summary of the conceptualization, assessing both cognitive and behavioral factors that influence the development of symptoms from both longitudinal and cross-sectional perspectives. The longitudinal conceptualization outlines how developmental processes and family relationships contributed to schema formation and how this led to the triggering of the symptoms. The cross-sectional conceptualization assesses how the triggering and sustaining factors are influencing the patient's automatic thoughts, mood, and behavior.

When setting treatment goals, it is important to distinguish between general and specific goals. General goals represent broader, future-oriented objectives, while specific goals are the concrete steps needed to achieve these overarching objectives. When setting goals, the therapist considers whether the goals are meaningful to the patient, within their control, and whether they are specific and realistic.

Finally, the treatment plan is developed based on the information gathered, detailing the specific methods to be used in CBT, pharmacotherapy, and environmental adjustments.

The process of conceptualization does not end once it has been created. If therapy is not progressing as expected, revising the conceptualization should be considered. As therapy continues, newly acquired findings and information are incorporated into the conceptualization, ensuring it remains a useful guide for the patient in front of you.

8 Neural Basis of Cognitive Behavioral Therapy

In the section on the cognitive behavioral model, it was mentioned that "CBT focuses on optimizing the collection of information for rapid cognition." But what neural basis underlies this process?

Diffusion tensor imaging (DTI) allows us to calculate the anisotropy of white matter nerve fibers as fractional anisotropy (FA) values. In essence, when nerve fibers run in a straight line, the FA value approaches 1, while disruptions in the fiber pathways result in a decrease in FA values. We conducted a study comparing DTI images of patients with mood disorders, including depression, to those of healthy individuals and reported a decrease in FA values in the white matter of the patient group [4]. White matter nerve fibers are insulated by myelin, which is produced by differentiated oligodendrocytes. We hypothesize that as mood disorders progress, abnormalities in the differentiation of oligodendrocytes disrupt myelin formation, causing disorganization in nerve fiber pathways, leading to a reduction in FA values. Our next area of interest is how treatment affects these microstructural brain changes caused by mood disorders.

To investigate this, we analyzed DTI images before and after 16 sessions of CBT, administered to 13 patients with depression as prescribed by the Ministry of Health, Labour, and Welfare. The average QIDS (Quick Inventory of Depressive Symptomatology) score for these 13 patients improved from 12.8 before treatment to 9.8 after treatment, indicating symptom improvement. As shown in Fig. 3, post-treatment FA value increases were observed in regions such as the cingulum, cerebellar vermis, external capsule, corpus callosum, and structures like the stria terminalis and fornix. This suggests that CBT helped correct disorganized nerve pathways and brain microstructural changes. Additionally, the FA improvements were more pronounced in the left hemisphere.

Which areas of the brain, related to this neural basis, are responsible for the improvements seen with CBT? The corpus callosum, particularly the anterior part, is involved in functional connections between the left and right frontal hemispheres. Improvement in the microstructural integrity of this region suggests enhanced functioning of the internal and external information processing systems. The external capsule is involved in the collection and processing of external information, and its improvement indicates an increase in functional connectivity between the posterior cortical areas and the frontal lobe, leading to more efficient external information processing systems. Improvements in the cingulum's microstructure suggest increased functional connectivity between the hippocampus and the frontal

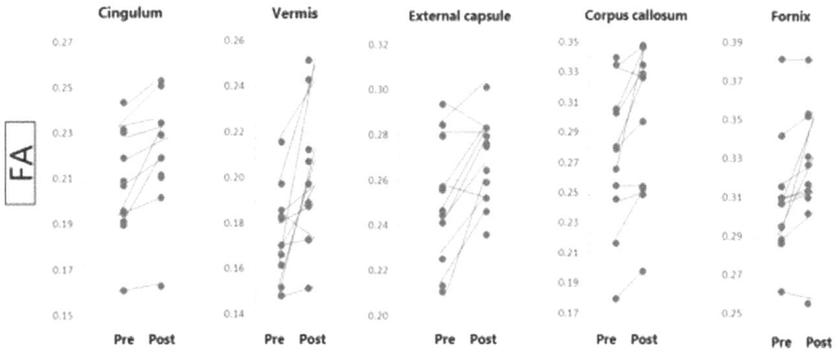

Fig. 3 .

lobe, which are involved in memory-related internal information, leading to the enhancement and activation of the internal information processing system.

Furthermore, improvements in the stria terminalis and cerebellar vermis suggest increased efficiency and activation in emotional processing systems, while improvements in the fornix indicate strengthened functional connections between the emotional and internal information processing systems. These findings suggest that strengthening the connections between four systems—the "internal and external information processing system," the "external information collection and processing system," the "internal information accumulation (memory)," and the "emotional processing system"—leads to symptom improvement. Additionally, the more pronounced increase in FA values in the left hemisphere suggests that CBT, which involves verbal communication, enhances, and strengthens the functional connectivity and activation of these systems.

These results collectively indicate that CBT's mechanism of action lies in the activation of information processing systems in the brain.

9 Conclusion

As discussed above, considering that "the target of Cognitive Behavioral Therapy (CBT) is the activation of information processing systems," there is potential for automating CBT using technologies such as AI.

References

1. M.E. Weishaar (Supervised by Yu Oono). *Aaron T. Beck: The Emergence and Evolution of Cognitive Therapy* (Tokyo: Sogensha, 2009), pp. 46–47

2. M.E. Weishaar (Supervised by Yu Oono). *Aaron T. Beck: The Emergence and Evolution of Cognitive Therapy* (Tokyo: Sogensha, 2009), pp. 42–44
3. M.E. Weishaar (Supervised by Yu Oono). *Aaron T. Beck: The Emergence and Evolution of Cognitive Therapy*. (Tokyo: Sogensha, 2009), pp. 57–60
4. K. Matsuoka, F. Yasuno, T. Kishimoto, A. Yamamoto, K. Kiuchi, J. Kosaka, K. Nagatsuka, H. Iida, T. Kudo, Microstructural differences in the corpus callosum in patients with bipolar disorder and major depressive disorder. J. Clin. Psychiatry **78**(1), 99–104 (2017)

Introduces the Measurement of Social Skills

Social Performance Rating

Jennifer Hamet Bagnou, Céline Clavel, Jean-Claude Martin, and Elise Prigent

Abstract Behavioral observation scales are important for understanding and assessing social skills. In this chapter, we explore tools for assessing social skills. It highlights the limitations of existing methods, such as self-assessments and observation tools, which often suffer from response bias. The chapter introduces and validates two scales: the SSC (Social Skill for Collaboration) for measuring collaborative problem-solving skills and the SPRS (Social Performance Rating Scale) for communication skills.

1 Introduction

Although social competence can be operationalized in different ways, it is conceptualized in the models previously discussed in Chap. 2 as an evaluative construct that refers to the judgments made by significant individuals within an individual's environment [1–3]. Consequently, to gain insight into an individual's social competence, assessment tools have been developed to capture observable behaviors and infer social performance.

In this chapter, we describe two scales for assessing social skills in human–human. We will begin by presenting the different existing methods and tools for measuring social skills. Then, we will present an example of scale validation in the context of collaborative problem-solving skills.

J. Hamet Bagnou (✉) · C. Clavel · J.-C. Martin · E. Prigent
Interdisciplinary Laboratory of Digital Sciences (LISN), Cognition, Perception and Uses Team, CNRS, Université Paris Saclay, Orsay, France
e-mail: hamet@lisn.fr

S. Nakamura (ed.), *Multimodal Interaction Technologies for Training Affective Social Skills*, https://doi.org/10.1007/978-981-96-1313-7_5

2 Methods and Tools for Measuring Social Skills

2.1 General Approach

Three main approaches are commonly used to assess social performance, a crucial aspect of social skills. These approaches are distinguished by their respective focus on the rate of social interaction, the performance of specific socially competent behaviors, or the adequacy of performance in meeting the demands of relevant social tasks [1, 3–8].

The approach based on the *rate of social interaction* measures the frequency of interactions with peers, a method initially popularized by Foster and Ritchey [9]. This method, particularly used with children, assumes that the number of interactions could reflect social performance. However, research has revealed significant limitations to this approach. Notably, the rate of interaction is not always positively correlated with indicators of social competence, such as sociometric status. For example, an individual may have a high number of interactions, but if these are marked by negative or aggressive behaviors, this rather indicates deficits in social performance [10, 11]. Consequently, this approach is increasingly less used in contemporary assessments due to its lack of sensitivity to the quality of social interactions [5].

The second approach focuses on the observation and evaluation of *specific behaviors* considered as indicators of social performance. These behaviors include prosocial acts such as giving compliments, assertiveness, or cooperative play, which can be observed in various social interactions [12–14]. This method allows for a fine-grained assessment of social skills through direct observation, self-assessments, or evaluations by peers, teachers, or parents. Although this approach seems theoretically valid, it has drawn criticism concerning its lack of empirical validity [3, 5, 9, 15, 16].

The third approach, considered more promising by several researchers, focuses on evaluating the adequacy of *performance in specific social tasks* [5, 7]. This method involves assessing the extent to which an individual effectively meets the demands of given social situations. This can be done either in a single situation with well-defined task criteria or in a broad range of more complex situations [3]. For example, an individual's ability to interact with a colleague in a professional setting could be evaluated based on specific criteria such as respecting interpersonal space or conflict resolution. This approach is particularly valued for its ability to adjust to the specifics of social interactions and to offer a more contextual measure of social competence [5, 7].

2.2 Behavioral Analyses

The behavioral approach constitutes an extension of the general approaches to evaluating social skills. It relies on expert judgments to assess social performance based on observed behavioral responses in specific situations [7, 17].

The first step of the behavioral analysis model involves identifying the critical situations that the target population is likely to encounter. This step is essential because it defines the framework within which social skills will be evaluated. The identified situations should be frequent, perceived as difficult, or require active problem-solving. Methods for identifying these situations are varied: direct observation of behavior, self-monitoring (e.g., diaries), surveys, or identification by significant others such as parents, teachers, or partners [5]. This step echoes the approach of performance adequacy in relevant social tasks discussed earlier, where identifying critical situations helps determine the context in which social competence can be meaningfully evaluated.

Once the key social situations are identified, the next step is to list possible responses and evaluate their effectiveness. Experts judge these responses based on their ability to resolve problematic situations while avoiding negative consequences [17]. This step allows for a contextual evaluation of social performance, similar to the performance adequacy approach previously discussed.

The evaluation of responses, the third step of the model, relies on expert judgments. These judgments are based on the definition of effectiveness proposed by Goldfried and D'Zurilla, stating that responses must "resolve the problematic nature of the situation and avoid potential negative consequences" [17]. The evaluation is thus intrinsically linked to the individual's ability to navigate effectively in complex social situations.

The final step of behavioral analysis involves developing specific measures to assess social performance. Ideally, these measures would rely on direct observation of behaviors in the identified critical situations. However, when direct observation is not possible, alternatives such as role-playing, imagined role-playing, or self-monitoring can be used [7]. These methods allow for capturing a variety of behaviors in controlled or semi-controlled contexts, and the responses can then be judged on their ability to effectively resolve problematic situations while minimizing negative consequences and maximizing positive outcomes.

Behavioral analysis not only allows for evaluating social performance but also for identifying moderating variables, such as psychological and demographic factors, that can influence social functioning [2].

3 Application of Tools for Measuring Social Competence to Collaborative Problem-Solving

During everyday interactions, social skills are often used along with other skills such as cognitive or motor skills. It is thus important to rate social performance in such situations.

Collaborative Problem-Solving (CPS) is a form of interaction that significantly contributes to the smooth functioning of a group or organization [18]. It is defined as a set of social skills jointly used to solve problems and work toward a common goal while socially collaborating with one another in a group of individuals [19–21]. Thus, CPS depends on individuals' ability to establish common ground regarding the nature of the problem, develop a solution plan, monitor progress along the way, and consider multiple viewpoints while respectfully managing disagreements. This requires the ability to understand the goals and constraints of the task, to take into account others' perspectives and knowledge, and the ability to communicate this understanding through negotiation, mutual regulation, and shared responsibility [22].

Recent research has identified CPS skills as essential for academic and professional success [23]. Indeed, as individuals enter the workforce, they are expected to work with others to solve complex and non-automatable problems, make decisions, and generate new ideas, which requires skills associated with CPS. Even experienced workers collaborate with their colleagues to combine their expertise and find a common solution to a problem.

Beyond work or studies, we also collaborate with others to solve different types of problems in our private lives, whether with our families, friends, or even strangers. If we look around us, almost all the objects surrounding us are the product of collaboration [24]. Their production extends to many fields such as entertainment, health, or engineering, which is evidence of the necessity of collaboration for progress and development [22, 24, 25].

All these areas require individuals to master problem-solving skills and social collaboration skills [20, 21], 26]. Difficulties in these social skills can therefore create social dysfunction, resulting in difficult social interactions with others, social withdrawal, and emotional distress [27]. These dysfunctions are often associated with the absence of the required skills, not using them in a timely manner, or when the individual adopts socially inappropriate behaviors [15, 27, 28], or with individual characteristics [25, 29], such as the level of anxiety [29, 30] or alexithymia [31].

Yet, as observed by Hesse and his collaborators [20], these complex skills useful during CPS tasks are neither formally taught nor evaluated. This is notably explained by the lack of consensus on a CPS model allowing for operationalizing this construct and measuring it [22, 23, 25].

Drawing inspiration from the general approaches and behavioral analysis discussed previously, assessment tools for CPS skills rely on several methods, such as self-assessments, situational judgment tests (SJTs), and tasks based on simulated scenarios. These tools are applied in various domains like business, education, healthcare, and the military sector.

Self-assessments, such as the VIEW scale (Creative Problem-Solving Group) [32] or the Tailored Adaptive Personality Assessment System (TAPAS) [33], are widely used to measure CPS skills using Likert scales or forced-choice questions. These tools, while attractive for their simplicity and low cost, present limitations similar to those observed in the evaluation of general social skills [19, 34]. Indeed, self-assessments are vulnerable to response biases, such as social desirability or the halo effect, and heavily depend on individuals' ability to self-evaluate accurately [34]. Continuing the criticisms directed at the approach of evaluating specific social behaviors, self-assessments may lack empirical validity because they rely on participants' subjective interpretation rather than on objective observations of behavior in real situations [35, 36] (ETS, 2012; OECD, 2012).

Situational Judgment Tests (SJTs), such as the Teamwork-KSA Test [25, 37], constitute a more contextual method for evaluating CPS skills. These tests present scenarios simulating real teamwork situations and ask participants to provide judgments or solutions. This approach is in direct connection with the behavioral analysis discussed earlier, where the effectiveness of responses is evaluated based on their adequacy in resolving specific social situations. SJTs are particularly useful for detecting subtle judgment processes and for engaging participants in realistic situations while maintaining some control over experimental variables [25, 38]. However, as with behavioral evaluation, SJTs can suffer from divergences between participants' evaluations and those of the experimenters, which can undermine the reliability of the results [25].

Tasks based on simulated scenarios offer an opportunity to directly observe participants' behaviors in controlled contexts. This method closely resembles the direct observation used in behavioral analysis, allowing for a more authentic evaluation of CPS skills. Participants are placed in simulated situations where they must interact with real or virtual teammates, which enables the capture of data on specific behaviors and their effectiveness. These tasks are often used in specific fields, such as health or medicine, where observing behaviors in critical situations is essential. For example, the University of Texas Behavioral Markers Audit Form [39] is used to evaluate teamwork skills during neonatal resuscitation simulations [25]. However, despite their realism and engagement, these tasks can still be subject to biases, notably when participants attempt to "manipulate" the results based on what they believe are the desired responses.

Assessment tools for CPS skills draw directly from the methods of evaluating social competence discussed in previous sections. They attempt to capture the complexity of collaborative interactions using approaches that combine observations, contextualization, and expert judgment [25].

However, although existing tools for evaluating CPS skills are diverse, they remain highly specific to certain domains, such as the military or medicine, and are not always transferable to other professional or personal contexts. They also present psychometric limitations that question their general validity and reliability. As observed in the general and behavioral approaches to evaluating social skills, this underscores the need to develop more robust assessment instruments that can be effectively applied to various contexts and populations.

In the sections below, we describe two scales for measuring different dimensions of social performance during CPS. We also explain the methodology for designing these two scales and illustrate their translation and application to the French language.

3.1 Design of Initial Items

The Assessment and Teaching of 21st Century Skills (ATC21S) project provides a basic set of items for rating social performance during CPS [35]. This framework is founded on the distinction between two very broad classes of skills: social skills and cognitive skills. Social skills constitute the "collaborative" dimension of collaborative problem-solving, while cognitive skills constitute the "problem-solving" dimension of collaborative problem-solving.

In the "problem-solving" dimension of CPS, group members work together to develop a common understanding of the problematic situation, exchange information, discuss the most appropriate strategies to solve the problem, monitor and revise their strategies until the group's objectives are achieved [40–42]. Indicators of these skills can be summarized under two headings: task regulation and knowledge building. Task regulation refers to learners' ability to set goals, manage resources, analyze and organize the problem space, explore a problem systematically, gather information, and tolerate ambiguity. Knowledge building concerns the individual's ability to understand the problem and test hypotheses.

The "collaborative" dimension includes communication processes among team members that can either facilitate or hinder problem-solving [43]. Participation, perspective-taking, argumentation, negotiation, and emotional and motivational interaction are examples of these communicative processes [20, 42]. Participation is the foundation of engagement with the task and other collaborators and is reflected in how people act or interact to accomplish tasks. Perspective-taking skills emphasize the quality of interaction among participants, reflecting their level of awareness of their collaborators' knowledge and resources as well as their responsiveness. Social regulation refers to the strategies used during collaboration, such as negotiation, initiative-taking, self-evaluation, and taking responsibility.

Thus, we obtain an initial annotation grid composed of 18 items divided into five domains (three for the social collaborative dimension and two for the problem-solving dimension; see Table 1). We find, for example, items evaluating the level of interaction, adaptation of discourse to others, and formulation of steps in problem-solving. Each item is evaluated on a scale ranging from 0 (low) to 2 (high).

Unlike other existing models, the one proposed by the ATC21S project lends itself more to the evaluation of human–human interaction and details the sub-skills of collaboration and problem-solving. It is also adaptable to several contexts [20, 21].

The complexity of CPS requires, in addition to the skills mentioned above, being attentive to the verbal and non-verbal communication skills of social partners (e.g., eye contact, voice quality, etc.). The individual must indeed decide which information is essential to react, develop a plan, rely on their repertoire of verbal and non-verbal skills, and implement it.

The Social Performance Rating Scale (SPRS) by Fydrich [30, 44, 45] allows for a qualitative evaluation of five items of communication skills within the framework of a multimodal social interaction. To account for the level of social skills mobilized during social interaction, the authors consider five categories of indicators.

Table 1 Social and cognitive skills in collaborative problem-solving, according to ATC21S [20]

Sub-dimension	Element	Description
"Collaborative" dimension		
Participation	Action	Activity within the environment
	Interaction	Interacting with, prompting, and responding to the contribution of others
	Task completion/ perseverance	Undertaking and completing a task or part of a task individually
Perspective taking	Adaptive responsiveness	Ignoring, accepting, or adapting to the contributions of others
	Audience awareness	Awareness of how to adapt behavior to increase suitability for others
Social regulation	Negotiation	Achieving a resolution or reaching a compromise
	Self-evaluation	Recognizing own strengths and weaknesses
	Transactive memory	Recognizing strengths and weaknesses of others
	Responsibility initiative	Assuming responsibility for ensuring part of the task are completed by the group
"Problem-solving" dimension		
Task regulation	Organizes	Analyses and describes a problem in familiar language
	Sets goals	Sets a clear goal for a task
	Resource management	Manages resources or people to complete a task
	Flexibility and ambiguity	Accepts ambiguous situations
	Collects elements of information	Explores and understands elements of the task
	Systematicity	Implements possible solutions to a problem and monitors progress
Learning and knowledge-building	Relationship	Identifies connections and patterns between and among elements of knowledge
	Rules "if… then"	Uses an understanding of cause and effect to develop a plan
	Hypothesis "what if…"	Adapts reasoning or course of action as information or circumstances change

The first indicator concerns the flow of the conversation, which requires approach behaviors toward a social partner, formulating a question or a statement, listening to the partner's response, maintaining the conversation, and ending the interaction [46–48]. Trower [49] observed that elements of conversation distinguished socially inadequate psychiatric patients from socially adequate ones [44]. In this item, a very low score will be attributed to a participant who makes few attempts to initiate the conversation, rarely uses open-ended questions, is intrusive in questioning, or shows no empathy.

The second indicator concerns voice quality (tone, pitch, clarity, volume). Indeed, a flat and monotone voice indicates a lack of social skills, whereas a voice deemed warm and enthusiastic reflects a high level of skill.

A third indicator concerns the length of phrases, that is, the rhythm/pressure of speech, speaking time, and pauses. Dow (1985) observed that "speaking time" and "pauses" were constant problems for socially anxious individuals in several social interactions. Indeed, monosyllabic speech ("hmmm," "yes," "OK") is associated with low social skills.

Gaze or eye contact is the fourth item on the SPRS scale. Associated with body orientation, gaze is linked to global evaluations of anxiety and skill among psychiatric patients [44, 50]. A participant who completely avoids looking at her partner or continually stares at them is judged as less socially proficient.

Finally, discomfort (fifth item) expressed during the interaction, for example through rigid body movements or facial tics, frequent throat clearing, inappropriate laughter, or sarcasm, can also indicate a low level of skill. Conversely, a relaxed posture and fluid gestures characterize high social skills.

The SPRS scale has been validated with a set of participants with anxiety disorders and therefore prone to difficulties in social interaction [44]. This scale is easily adaptable to all ages and a wide range of situations [51, 52]. The SPRS scale is short and easy to use, unlike other scales such as the Social Behavior Scale by Trower [53]. SPRS is applicable to the observation of conversations recorded on video or occurring live between two people. Observers are invited to evaluate behaviors on a five-point scale.

SPRS and the CPS are complementary from the point of view of evaluating social skills in that the CPS scale focuses on the skills involved in collaborative problem-solving, whereas the SPRS evaluates more general social skills, not specific to CPS but likely to facilitate it. They therefore allow for both general information on social interactions and specifics related to CPS.

3.2 Translation and Cross-Cultural Validation

In the following sections, we illustrate how we adapted and applied the two scales described above to measure social skills in French dyadic interactions during CPS. As suggested by Wild et al. (2005) in their guide to good practice in translation and cultural adaptation, an initial translation should be carried out from English to

French, followed by a back-translation from French to English. This forward–backward translation method provides quality control to verify the consistency between the translation and the original version. Each of the two scales was translated by Lionbridge (Dublin, Ireland), a company specializing in linguistic and intercultural adaptation.

3.3 Adaptation of the Scales

To verify the comprehensibility and to validate the content of the two annotation scales, we pre-tested them by annotating six participants (a total of 18 videos, one per collaborative game). The annotations were performed by four annotators, all experts in human behavior (two psychologists and two researchers in psychology and human–machine interaction).

We measured the inter-rater agreement using the intra-class correlation coefficient (ICC, 2 k). This coefficient defines the reliability of the evaluations by comparing the variability of the different evaluations of the same individual to the total variation of all evaluations and all individuals [54]. In our case, a sample of four evaluators was selected, and they evaluated all participants. We opted for the two-way random ICC with the mean as the unit of evaluation. Meetings between the evaluators allowed us to perform a qualitative validation of the content (comprehensibility, acceptability, response modality).

Regarding the CPS scale, the results indicated that the items of the "problem-solving" dimension, as well as the items "Self-evaluation" and "Transactive Memory" of the "collaborative" dimension, led to very low inter-rater agreements and "not applicable" responses.

These items were also considered by the annotators as the most difficult to understand and are specific to a type of CPS (e.g., tasks centered on problem-solving and not on collaboration). We therefore removed these items from the CPS scale.

Thus, we finally kept seven items: action, interaction, and perseverance for the sub-dimension Participation; adaptive responsiveness and audience awareness for the sub-dimension Perspective-Taking; and negotiation and responsibility/initiative for the sub-dimension Social Regulation (see Table 2).

We also reworked and expanded the wording of the remaining items to adapt them to three collaborative games (Table 3). For example, we defined the item "responsibility/initiative" as "the ability to take responsibility for working on a common representation of the problem, developing a strategic plan towards a solution, and monitoring the group's progress. This skill also includes asking questions, inquiring if the other has suggestions, acknowledging others' contributions, and helping to maintain team organization."

Initially, this item was defined as: "Assuming responsibility for ensuring parts of the task are completed by the group." Given that only the "collaborative" dimension remains from the original scale, we decided to name this revised scale it the "Social Skills of Collaboration Scale" (SSC).

Table 2 Adaptation of Social skills in collaborative problem-solving

Item	Description
"Collaborative" dimension	
Action	Refers to the skill of participating within the group, whether or not this action is coordinated with other group members The highest score will be given to participants who need very little guidance in the instructions to act in the problem-solving. They are comfortable in both familiar and unfamiliar situations
Interaction	Refers to the skill of engaging in verbal and non-verbal behaviors that demonstrate interaction with others The highest level of interaction skills is demonstrated if participants actively initiate coordination efforts, or prompt their collaborators to respond
Task completion/ perseverance	Refers to the skill of engaging in the task. The highest score will be given to participants who persist in engagement as indicated by multiple attempts at the problem or by trying different strategies
Adaptive responsiveness	Refers to the skill of integrating the contributions of collaborators into one's own thoughts and actions when solving a problem. Participants are able to integrate the contributions of collaborators into their own thoughts and actions. Individuals who rethink the representation of a problem based on evidence reported by a partner demonstrate a high degree of responsiveness
Audience awareness	Refers to the skill of adapting one's contributions to others by adapting one's words to the views of others or by making one's actions visible and understandable to others
Negotiation	Refers to the skill of reaching a resolution or compromise. The participant comments on the ideas of others, offers reasons to support or refute certain statements, negotiates in case of disagreement, and implements consensual solutions after discussion
Responsibility initiative	Refers to the skill of taking responsibility for working on a common representation of the problem, developing a strategic plan toward a solution, and monitoring the group's progress. This skill also includes asking questions, asking if the other has suggestions, acknowledging the contributions of others, and helping to keep the team organized

Finally, the four annotators reported difficulties with the scoring system ranging from 0 to 2, which did not allow for precise and discriminating evaluation of the skills. We therefore made the scoring system more quantitative and more homogeneous with the SPRS scale, moving from a rating of 0 to 2 to a rating of 1 to 5.

Following the preliminary results of the adaptation of the scales indicating good inter-rater agreement and consistency between the measurement items and the tasks for the SPRS scale, no structural changes were undertaken (see Table 3).

Table 3 Social performance rating scale, Fydrich, 1998

Item	Description
Gaze	(1) Very Poor: Participant completely avoids looking at the partner or stares continually (5) Very Good: Participant keeps eye contact during the conversation, does not stare or shifts focus during pauses and conversation
Vocal quality	(1) Very Poor: (a) Participant speaks in a flat, monotonous voice; or (b) speaks at a low volume or mumbles; or (c) speaks overly loudly, or has intrusive tone (harsh or unpleasant voice quality) (5) Very Good: Participant is warm and enthusiastic in verbal expression without sounding condescending or gushy
Conversation flow	(1) Very Poor: Participant makes few attempts to initiate the conversation. Even when prompted by the partner, participant cannot maintain the conversation. Participant uses almost no open-ended questions or is intrusive in questions and shows no empathy. Participant does not attend to information provided by the partner (5) Very Good: Participant easily maintains the conversation and responds smoothly to pauses in the conversation, often by following up on previous information provided by the partner or providing free information about the self on a related topic. Participant introduces new topics fluidly and frequently uses open-ended questions. Participant shows genuine interest in the partner and follows up on the partner's remarks with warmth or enthusiasm
Discomfort	(1) Very High: Complete rigidity of arms, legs, or whole body. Constant leg movements or fidgeting with hands, hair, or clothing. Extremely stiff face or constant facial tics. Frequent nervous throat clearing, swallowing, or stuttering. Frequent inappropriate giggling or laughing. Look of extreme discomfort and desire to flee the situation shown by 2 or more breaks in the role. Participant does not pay attention to the role-play tasks most of the time (5) Very Low: Relaxed body posture and natural body movement. Participant laughs and smiles at appropriate times. S/he shows effective gesturing (to be distinguished from fidgeting). Participant focuses on the task all the time, and does not appear at all uncomfortable, but at ease in the situation
Length	(1) Very Poor: Monosyllabic ('hmmm', 'yeah', 'OK') speech turns; or responses so long that the partner must interrupt or cannot utter a reply (5) Very Good: At most times, participant's utterances are two or more sentences long. Participant acknowledges partner's remarks without taking over and monopolizing the conversation

3.4 Validation Study: Human–Human Interaction

We conducted a psychometric evaluation of the revised scales. To this end, we assessed the internal consistency of each scale, the inter-rater reliability, and the structural validity using exploratory factor analysis. We measured convergent and divergent validity through correlations with measures of social anxiety and alexithymia, which have been observed to impact performance in social interactions [44, 55].

3.4.1 Participants

We recruited 76 participants randomly assigned to 38 dyads. Recruitment was carried out within the general population through advertisements on websites and within the University. Eligible individuals were at least 18 years old, without language disorders, and fluent in French.

3.4.2 Protocol

Upon recruitment, participants completed questionnaires via the online platform Limesurvey (www.limesurvey.org). These questionnaires allowed us to collect information regarding the participants' individual characteristics, such as the types of difficulties they experience or their emotional states. These questionnaires will be discussed in more detail in the "Measures" section.

Once the questionnaires were completed, participants were randomly assigned into pairs and invited to the laboratory to perform collaborative games. These are the three collaborative games presented in the "Corpus" section: "Prisoner's Dilemma," "Survival Task," and "Invest for the University." The interaction took place via a videoconferencing platform without any support other than video.

Participants received the following general instruction: "During each game, you will need to discuss together and collaborate to find a common solution to each of the problems presented to you." The experimenter specified to the participants that their conversation would not be listened to and that they could exchange freely.

3.4.3 Measures

The SSC and SPRS annotation scales are provided in the Appendices. In order to enable us to study the impact of individual differences on social skills during collaborative problem-solving games, we asked participants to complete self-report questionnaires before performing the three collaborative tasks.

The Toronto Alexithymia Scale (TAS-20) [56] is the most commonly used scale to assess alexithymia. This scale consists of 20 items divided into three dimensions: difficulty identifying emotions, difficulty describing emotions, and externally-oriented thinking. Responses are rated from 1 "strongly disagree" to 5 "strongly agree."

The Social Interaction Anxiety Scale (SIAS) [57] assesses anxiety related to social interactions, defined as extreme distress when initiating and maintaining conversations with friends, strangers, or potential partners. It comprises 20 items rated from 0 "not at all characteristic of me" to 4 "extremely characteristic of me."

The Beck Depression Inventory (BDI) [58, 59] evaluates the presence of depressive symptoms in participants. This scale consists of 13 items rated from 0 to 3. The higher the score, the more severe the depressive symptoms.

3.4.4 Annotators and Annotation Procedure

The annotators were previously introduced to the protocol and the two scales. Among them, two are trained in psychology, one is a clinical psychologist, and the last annotator is an expert in Human–Machine Interaction. They received annotation training and participated in the modifications made to the scales. During this training phase, the evaluations of each collaborative game were discussed, and divergences were resolved. To ensure cohesion and common understanding of the items, the evaluators met after each annotation to jointly review the interaction videos, discuss discrepancies between the original evaluations, and justify their annotations.

To perform their annotations, the annotators received the scales in the form of an Excel spreadsheet with the following instructions: "You will watch videos depicting interactions between two people (one video for each game). After each video, you must evaluate each participant's social performance. Please note that you must watch the video at least twice before starting your evaluation. Once the evaluation is completed, you must watch the video again at least once before you can definitively validate your responses."

3.4.5 Statistical Analysis

Analyses were performed on the mean scores of the three games. A repeated-measures ANOVA showed no significant effect of the game on the scores of each item (all $p > 0.05$). Consequently, the annotation scores were averaged over the three role-playing games performed by each subject to obtain a more reliable assessment of social performance.

The psychometric analysis included the evaluation of item characteristics of the SSC and SPRS scales, construct validity, internal consistency, and convergent and divergent validity.

Spearman correlation coefficients (rs) were calculated to examine the homogeneity of the scale (item-total correlation, with a minimum acceptable level of $rs > 0.3$) and to identify if highly correlated items should be omitted due to redundancy (inter-item correlations, $rs > 0.9$). A correlation network graph was constructed from these results to graphically illustrate the relationships between items (see Fig. 2B for the SSC scale and 4B for SPRS).

The construct validity (factor structure) of the scales was evaluated using exploratory factor analysis (principal factor method with non-orthogonal oblique rotation, also known as oblimin rotation; [60]) to examine the underlying constructs and characterize dimensionality. Data were first examined using Bartlett's test of sphericity ($p < 0.001$ for both scales) and the Kaiser–Meyer–Olkin (KMO) measure of sampling adequacy (for SSC = 0.90; for SPRS = 0.86), indicating that our sample was appropriate for conducting Exploratory Factor Analyses (EFA; [61]). We used various strategies to determine the optimal number of factors to retain, including considering the proportion of variance explained for the retained factor solution, using Horn's parallel analysis (Horn, 1965) based on the 95th percentile estimate,

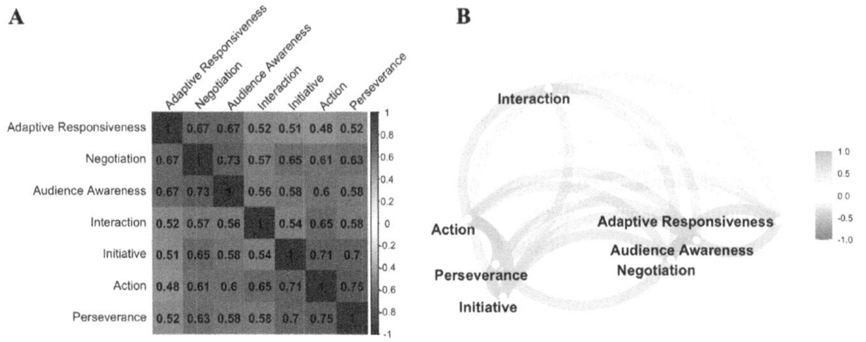

Fig. 1 Correlation Between Items—(A) Spearman's Rank Correlation Coefficient Matrix and (B) Correlation Network. The matrix contains Spearman's rank correlation coefficients between the seven items of the SSC questionnaire. Colors indicate the direction and strength of the correlation, with positive correlations displayed in blue and negative correlations in red. Results in bold indicate statistical significance at the $p < 0.05$ level. The correlation network is constructed from all pairwise correlations between the items in (A). Items are represented by nodes and connected by edges. Red and blue lines represent negative and positive correlations, respectively. The saturation of the color and the width of the lines are proportional to the strength of the correlation

and calculating Velicer's Minimum Average Partial (MAP) criterion [62]. Finally, items were considered for deletion if their factor loadings were < 0.4 and/or if their communalities were < 0.3 (uniqueness > 0.7).

The reliability of internal consistency (item homogeneity) was assessed by calculating Cronbach's alpha coefficient [63]. A coefficient score > 0.8 indicates good internal consistency, and > 0.9 is considered excellent.

Finally, convergent validity was studied using Spearman correlations between the total sum of the items of each scale and an alexithymia scale. Divergent validity was measured using a correlation with a state anxiety scale and then with a social anxiety scale specific to social interaction.

Statistical analyses were performed using JASP software Version 0.16.1 (JASP Team, 2022, University of Amsterdam) for descriptive and factor analyses, and R 4.1.3 GUI 1.77 High Sierra build (R Foundation for Statistical Computing, Vienna, Austria) using the packages paran and psych for Horn's parallel analysis and Velicer's Minimum Average Partial correlation for determining the number of principal components, respectively.

3.4.6 Results

Factor Structure

We performed an inter-item Spearman correlation. The results indicate that all inter-item correlations are positive and significant (Fig. 1 for SSC correlation). The item with the lowest correlation is the "action" item.

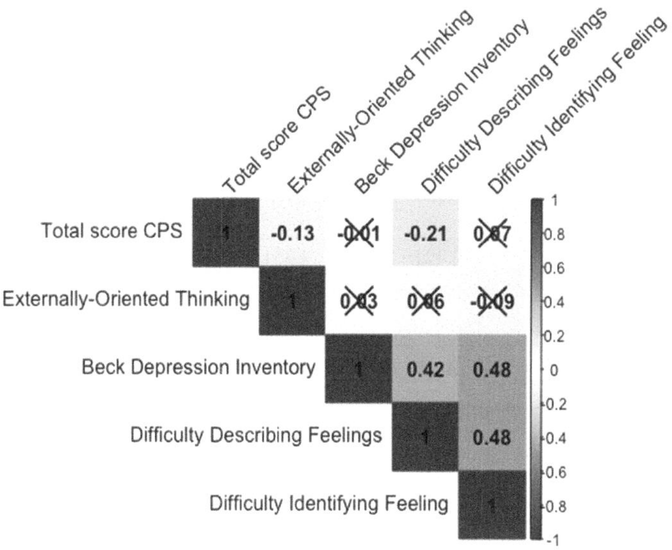

Fig. 2 Correlation indicating SSC convergent and divergent validity. Non-significant correlations are marked with an X

An exploratory factor analysis was performed on the seven items of the SSC scale using oblique rotation (oblimin). The one-factor solution had eigenvalues exceeding Kaiser's criterion of 1 and explained 65.4% of the variance. The scree plot was slightly ambiguous and showed inflections that would justify retaining both one and two factors. Given the sample size and the convergence of the scree plot and Kaiser's criterion on one factor, the one-factor solution was retained in the final analysis.

We observe that all items have factor loadings ranging between 0.738 and 0.854. Table 4 also displays the 'uniqueness' of each variable. Uniqueness represents the proportion of variance that is specific to the variable and not explained by the factor. The greater the uniqueness, the lower the relevance or saturation of the variable within the factor model. For example, 45.6% of the variance of the item 'Adaptive Responsiveness' is not explained by the one-factor solution. In contrast, the uniqueness of the item 'Action' is relatively low, with only 27% of its variance not accounted for by the factor solution.

Thus, the factor analysis of the SSC scale identifies a single factor (or domain) comprising seven items. This factor is related to collaboration and describes the entire set of social skills necessary for its execution.

The Spearman correlation conducted between the five items of the SPRS also yielded significant results and positive relationships.

The five SPRS items were also subjected to an exploratory factor analysis (EFA) using an oblique rotation (oblimin). For reasons similar to those for the SSC scale, a single-factor solution was favored over a two-factor solution. This single-factor solution explains 67.1% of the variance. Factor loadings ranged from 0.72 for the "gaze" item to 0.88 for the "length" item. The factor analysis identified one factor

Table 4 SSC's factor loading

Item	Factor 1	Uniqueness	Mean	Std.	S	K
Adaptive responsiveness	0.738	0.456	4.303	0.587	−0.893	0.878
Negotiation	0.834	0.305	4.216	0.634	−0.756	0.038
Audience awareness	0.796	0.367	4.194	0.645	−0.714	0.129
Interaction	0.761	0.421	4.351	0.720	−1.303	1.540
Initiative	0.837	0.299	4.376	0.665	−1.129	0.857
Action	0.854	0.270	4.592	0.579	−1.684	2.922
Perseverance	0.836	0.300	4.375	0.683	−1.007	0.442

Std.: Standard deviation; S: Skewness; K: Kurtosis

composed of five items. This factor corresponds to verbal and non-verbal social skills required in the context of communication with others.

3.4.7 Reliability

For the scale validation, inter-rater reliability was measured by calculating the intra-class correlation coefficient (ICC, 2 k). This coefficient defines the reliability of ratings by comparing the variability of different ratings of the same individual to the total variation across all ratings and individuals (Shrout and Fleiss, 1979). In our case, the videos were annotated by at least two raters. Therefore, we employed a two-way random effects model ICC with the average as the unit of evaluation.

The intra-class correlation coefficient ranges from 0 to 1. The results indicate reliability ranging from moderate to excellent for the items across both scales. Values below 0.5 indicate poor reliability, values between 0.5 and 0.75 indicate moderate reliability, values between 0.75 and 0.9 indicate good reliability, and values above 0.9 indicate excellent reliability [64].

For the SSC scale, all items showed moderate to good reliability (ranging from 0.54 for the item "Adaptive Responsiveness" to 0.80 for the item "Interaction"; see Table 5).

For the SPRS scale, all items demonstrated moderate to good reliability, except for the "Discomfort" item, which showed poor reliability (0.50).

3.4.8 Internal Consistency, Convergent, and Divergent Validity

A measure of overall performance was created by summing the raw scores of the seven items. This measure demonstrated excellent internal consistency (Cronbach's alpha = 0.928; McDonald's omega = 0.929).

Table 5 Inter-rater reliability for the SSC scale

Item	ICC 2 K
Adaptive responsiveness	0.54
Negotiation	0.62
Audience awareness	0.66
Interaction	0.80
Initiative	0.70
Action	0.69
Perseverance	0.65

Spearman correlations were calculated between the total score and questionnaire measures (Fig. 2). Good convergent validity was demonstrated by moderate to strong correlations between the total score on the SSC scale and the alexithymia dimensions "Difficulty Describing Feelings" (TAS DDF, $r = -0.21$, $p = 0.001$) and "Externally-Oriented Thinking" (EOT, $r = -0.13$, $p = 0.05$). This indicates that higher scores in these dimensions are associated with lower performance in social skills and collaboration. For divergent validity, a weak correlation between the SSC scale and the depression scale (BDI) was found ($r = -0.01$, $p = 0.83$).

A similar approach was applied to the SPRS scale. The scale showed excellent internal consistency (Cronbach's alpha = 0.902; McDonald's omega = 0.901), which is higher than that reported by Fydrich et al. [44] during the scale's construction.

Spearman correlations were also calculated between the total score on the SPRS scale and the alexithymia scale scores. Good convergent validity was again demonstrated by moderate to strong correlations between the SPRS and the alexithymia measures (EOT, $r = -0.20$, $p < 0.001$; DDF, $r = -0.26$, $p < 0.001$). Participants with higher alexithymia scores showed lower performance ratings.

Regarding divergent validity, we again found a weak correlation between the SPRS scale and the Beck Depression Inventory (BDI) scale ($r = 0.05$, $p = 0.15$; not significant).

4 Conclusion

Current tools for evaluating social skills, such as self-assessments (e.g., the VIEW scale, Creative Problem-Solving Group, 2013 [32]), situational judgment tests (e.g., The Teamwork-KSA Test) [37], and third-party evaluations or observation tools, present numerous limitations. Self-assessment methods (using forced-choice or Likert scales) and situational judgment tests have a high risk of response bias (social desirability, extreme responses, acquiescence, halo effect). Moreover, these tools require participants to possess high metacognitive abilities to judge their own level of performance. They can also lead to discrepancies between the experimenter's judgment and that of the participant. Regarding third-party evaluations, existing observation tools are often limited to the fields of health and medicine (e.g., the Communication and Teamwork Skills assessment) [11] and the military domain (Anti-Air Teamwork Observation Measure)[65]. Several scales have been developed for assessing Human-Agent (chatbot) interactions rather than between two humans [21, 66]. Additionally, their psychometric analyses show low inter-rater reliability [25].

Finally, these tools are often used in the context of admission to higher education and aim at young participants transitioning from one educational level to another [25]. However, Collaborative Problem-Solving (CPS) skills are acquired throughout life, and even experienced workers must collaborate with their colleagues to combine their expertise and find a common solution to a problem [21, 26].

Therefore, it is essential to develop and validate qualitative measurement instruments of social performance that are adaptable to different situations and free from response biases, thus allowing for an adequate evaluation of social skill [21, 66]. In this chapter, we explained how we collected a new corpus of videos featuring dyadic collaborative interactions and validated two scales that enable the evaluation of social skills.

We developed the SSC scale based on items derived from existing inventories of collaborative problem-solving skills (Hesse et al., 2015). These inventories were refined by experts in human behavior, and seven items were selected and reformulated due to their relevance in a collaborative interaction context.

The SPRS scale is designed to evaluate social skills related to communication during social interactions. The English version was translated and adapted to French. Apart from the translation, no modifications were made to the original version, as it was considered suitable for collaborative interaction contexts.

These two scales measure distinct yet complementary constructs. While the SSC scale assesses skills specific to the context of collaboration, the SPRS scale evaluates general multimodal communication skills, which are prerequisites for collaboration skills.

Psychometric analyses confirmed that SSC and SPRS scales are valid and reliable instruments for measuring social skills. Factor analysis revealed a one-factor solution for each scale, explaining over 65% of the variance for the SSC and 67% for the SPRS. Reliability coefficients from the psychometric analysis indicated excellent internal consistency (0.93 for the SSC and 0.90 for the SPRS). Unlike existing tools [19, 25], our two scales exhibited moderate to good inter-rater reliability.

The convergent and divergent validity of SPRS and SSC were confirmed by the pattern of correlations with other reliable and valid measures: correlations with measures of alexithymia (difficulty identifying emotions and externally-oriented thinking) were significant, whereas those with measures of depression were not. These results are consistent with those highlighted by Fydrich [44] during the development of the SPRS scale. According to the literature on social skills training [15, 25], these findings are of particular interest since the development of collaborative problem-solving skills has been defined as essential for professional, academic, and personal success. Their evaluation with reliable and valid instruments would allow training sessions to be targeted at individuals' difficulties as well as according to their profile (e.g., alexithymic or anxious individuals). It would also be possible to monitor participants' progress throughout social skills training and thus verify its effectiveness. Other research (see Chapter 6 in this book) has replicated this validation within the Japanese population and in other interaction contexts, demonstrating that the SSC and SPRS scales can be useful to a wide range of researchers interested in evaluating social skills.

References

1. F.M. Gresham, G. Sugai, R.H. Horner, Interpreting outcomes of social skills training for students with high-incidence disabilities. Except. Child. **67**(3), 331–344 (2001). https://doi.org/10.1177/001440290106700303
2. M.A. Dirks, T.A. Treat, V.R. Weersing, The situation specificity of youth responses to peer provocation. J. Clin. Child Adolesc. Psychol. **36**(4), 621–628 (2007). https://doi.org/10.1080/15374410701662758
3. R.M. McFall, A review and reformulation of the concept of social skills. Behav. Assess. **4**(1), 1–33 (1982). https://doi.org/10.1007/BF01321377
4. S.R. Asher, An evolving paradigm in social skill training research with children, in *Children's Peer Relations: Issues in Assessment and Intervention*, B.H. Schneider, K.H. Rubin, and J.E. Ledingham, (eds.), (New York, NY: Springer US, 1985), pp. 157–171. https://doi.org/10.1007/978-1-4684-6325-5_10
5. T. Cavell, Social adjustment, social performance, and social skills: a tri-component model of social competence. J. Clin. Child Adolesc. Psychol. **19**(2), 111–122 (1990). https://doi.org/10.1207/s15374424jccp1902_2
6. F.M. Gresham, Conceptual and definitional issues in the assessment of children's social skills: Implications for classification and training. J. Clin. Child Psychol. **15**(1), 3–15 (1986). https://doi.org/10.1207/s15374424jccp1501_1
7. R.L. Grover, D.W. Nangle, M. Buffie, L.A. Andrews, Defining social skills, in *Social Skills Across the Life Span*, (Elsevier, 2020), pp. 3–24. https://doi.org/10.1016/B978-0-12-817752-5.00001-9
8. T. Hall, Review of experimental social behavioral interventions for preschool children: an evidenced-based synthesis. SAGE Open **10**(1), 2158244019899420 (2020). https://doi.org/10.1177/2158244019899420
9. S.L. Foster, W.L. Ritchey, Issues in the assessment of social competence in children. J. Appl. Behav. Anal. **12**(4), 625–638 (1979). https://doi.org/10.1901/jaba.1979.12-625
10. S.R. Asher, R.A. Markell, S. Hymel, Identifying children at risk in peer relations: a critique of the rate-of-interaction approach to assessment. Child Dev. **52**(4), 1239–1245 (1981). https://doi.org/10.2307/1129512
11. F.M. Gresham, Assessment of children's social skills. J. Sch. Psychol. **19**(2), 120–133 (1981). https://doi.org/10.1016/0022-4405(81)90054-6
12. E.S. Berler, A.M. Gross, R.S. Drabman, Social skills training with children: proceed with caution. J. Appl. Behav. Anal. **15**(1), 41–53 (1982). https://doi.org/10.1901/jaba.1982.15-41
13. L. Michelson, R. Wood, Behavioral assessment and training of children's social skills, in *Progress in Behavior Modification*, vol. 9, M. Hersen, R.M. Eisler, P.M. Miller, (eds.), (Elsevier, 1980), pp. 241–292. https://doi.org/10.1016/B978-0-12-535609-1.50012-X
14. S. Oden, S.R. Asher, Coaching children in social skills for friendship making. Child Dev. **48**(2), 495–506 (1977). https://doi.org/10.2307/1128645
15. A.S. Bellack, Recurrent problems in the behavioral assessment of social skill. Behav. Res. Ther. **21**(1), 29–41 (1983). https://doi.org/10.1016/0005-7967(83)90123-7

16. H. Hops, Children's social competence and skill: current research practices and future directions. Behav. Ther. **14**(1), 3–18 (1983). https://doi.org/10.1016/S0005-7894(83)80084-7
17. M.R. Goldfried, T.J. D'Zurilla A behavioral-analytic model for assessing competence1 1the preparation of this paper was supported by research grant mh-15044 from the united states public health service, national institute of mental health. The authors are grateful to Anita P. Goldfried, Ronald N. Kent, David M. Pomeranz, Charles D. Spielberger for their comments on an earlier version of the manuscript, in *Current Topics in Clinical and Community Psychology*, vol. 1, (C. D. Spielberger, Ed., Elsevier, 1969), pp. 151–196. https://doi.org/10.1016/B978-1-4831-9972-6.50009-3
18. J.D. Aram, C.P. Morgan, E.S. Esbeck, Relation of collaborative interpersonal relationships to individual satisfaction and organizational performance. Adm. Sci. Q. **16**(3), 289–297 (1971). https://doi.org/10.2307/2391901
19. H.O'Neil, S. Chuang, E. Baker, *Computer-Based Feedback for Computer-Based Collaborative Problem Solving*, (2010). https://doi.org/10.1007/978-1-4419-5662-0_14
20. F. Hesse, E. Care, J. Buder, K. Sassenberg, P. Griffin, A framework for teachable collaborative problem solving skills in *Assessment and teaching of 21st century skills educational assessment in an information age*, (2015), pp. 37–56. https://doi.org/10.1007/978-94-017-9395-7_2
21. M. Stadler, K. Herborn, M. Mustafić, S. Greiff, The assessment of collaborative problem solving in PISA 2015: an investigation of the validity of the PISA 2015 CPS tasks. Comput. Educ. **157**, 2020, https://doi.org/10.1016/j.compedu.2020.103964
22. C. Sun, V.J. Shute, A. Stewart, J. Yonehiro, N. Duran, S. D'Mello, Towards a generalized competency model of collaborative problem solving. Comput. Educ. **143**, 103672 (2020). https://doi.org/10.1016/j.compedu.2019.103672
23. J. Andrews-Todd, C. Forsyth, Exploring social and cognitive dimensions of collaborative problem solving in an open online simulation-based task. Comput. Hum. Behav. **104**, 105759 (2020). https://doi.org/10.1016/j.chb.2018.10.025
24. E. Hutchins, *Cognition in the Wild* (Bradford Books, Cambridge, MA, USA, 1995)
25. M.E. Oliveri, R. Lawless, H. Molloy, A literature review on collaborative problem solving for college and workforce readiness. ETS Res. Rep. Ser. **2017**(1), 1–27 (2017). https://doi.org/10.1002/ets2.12133
26. A.C. Graesser, S.M. Fiore, S. Greiff, J. Andrews-Todd, P.W. Foltz, F.W. Hesse, Advancing the science of collaborative problem solving. Psychol. Sci. Public Interest **19**(2), 59–92 (2018). https://doi.org/10.1177/1529100618808244
27. A.S. Bellack, Skills training for people with severe mental illness. Psychiatr. Rehabil. J. **27**(4), 375–391 (2004). https://doi.org/10.2975/27.2004.375.391
28. J.N. Kingery, C.A. Erdley, E. Scarpulla, Developing social skills, in *Social Skills Across the Life Span*, (Elsevier, 2020), pp. 25–45. https://doi.org/10.1016/B978-0-12-817752-5.00002-0.
29. J.O. Greene, B.R. Burleson, *Handbook of Communication and Social Interaction Skills* (Psychology Press, 2003)
30. S. Stevens et al., What determines observer-rated social performance in individuals with social anxiety disorder? J. Anxiety Disord. **24**(8), 830–836 (2010). https://doi.org/10.1016/j.janxdis.2010.06.005
31. C. Spitzer, U. Siebel-Jürges, S. Barnow, H.J. Grabe, H.J. Freyberger, Alexithymia and Interpersonal Problems. Psychother. Psychosom. **74**(4), 240–246 (2005). https://doi.org/10.1159/000085148
32. S.G. Isaksen, C. Hoßbach, VIEW: An assessment of problem-solving style—20 years of progress, Psychol. Rep. p. 00332941241249954, (2024). https://doi.org/10.1177/00332941241249954.
33. F. Drasgow, Intelligence and the workplace, in *Handbook of Psychology,* 2nd edn. (Wiley, 2012). https://doi.org/10.1002/9781118133880.hop212008
34. X. Zhuang, C. MacCann, L. Wang, L. Liu, R.D. Roberts, Development and validity evidence supporting a teamwork and collaboration assessment for high school students. ETS Res. Rep. Ser. **2008**(2), i–51 (2008). https://doi.org/10.1002/j.2333-8504.2008.tb02136.x

35. P. Griffin, E. Care, (eds.), *Assessment and Teaching of 21st Century Skills: Methods and Approach.* (Dordrecht: Springer Netherlands, 2015). https://doi.org/10.1007/978-94-017-9395-7
36. OECD, *Learning a Living: First Results of the Adult Literacy and Life Skills Survey.* Paris: Organisation for economic co-operation and development, (2005). https://www.oecd-ilibrary.org/education/learning-a-living_9789264010390-en. Accessed 07 Jun 2024
37. M.J. Stevens, M.A. Campion, Staffing work teams: development and validation of a selection test for teamwork settings. J. Manag. **25**(2), 207–228 (1999). https://doi.org/10.1016/S0149-2063(99)80010-5
38. J.A. Weekley, R.E. Ployhart, Eds., *Situational Judgment Tests: Theory, Measurement, and Application.* (New York: Psychology Press, 2005). https://doi.org/10.4324/9780203774878
39. E.J. Thomas, J.B. Sexton, R.L. Helmreich, Translating teamwork behaviours from aviation to healthcare: development of behavioural markers for neonatal resuscitation. BMJ Qual. Saf. **13**(suppl 1), i57–i64 (2004)
40. R.A. Baron, G.D. Markman, Beyond social capital: the role of entrepreneurs' social competence in their financial success. J. Bus. Ventur. **18**(1), 41–60 (2003). https://doi.org/10.1016/S0883-9026(00)00069-0
41. B. Zimmerman, D. Schunk, Self-regulated learning and performance: an introduction and an overview, Handb. Self-Regul. Learn. Perform. pp. 1–15, (2011)
42. B. Slof, D. Nijdam, J. Janssen, Do interpersonal skills and interpersonal perceptions predict student learning in CSCL-environments?, Comput. Educ. **97**, 2016, https://doi.org/10.1016/j.compedu.2016.02.012
43. J. Janssen, G. Erkens, P.A. Kirschner, G. Kanselaar, Task-related and social regulation during online collaborative learning. Metacognition Learn. **7**(1), 25–43 (2012). https://doi.org/10.1007/s11409-010-9061-5
44. T. Fydrich, D.L. Chambless, K.J. Perry, F. Buergener, M.B. Beazley, Behavioral assessment of social performance: a rating system for social phobia. Behav. Res. Ther. **36**(10), 995–1010 (1998). https://doi.org/10.1016/S0005-7967(98)00069-2
45. K. Ramdhonee-Dowlot, K. Balloo, C.A. Essau, Effectiveness of the super skills for life programme in enhancing the emotional wellbeing of children and adolescents in residential care institutions in a low- and middle-income country: a randomised waitlist-controlled trial. J. Affect. Disord. **278**, 327–338 (2021). https://doi.org/10.1016/j.jad.2020.09.053
46. W.H. Dotson, J.B. Leaf, J.B. Sheldon, J.A. Sherman, Group teaching of conversational skills to adolescents on the autism spectrum. Res. Autism Spectr. Disord. **4**(2), 199–209 (2010). https://doi.org/10.1016/j.rasd.2009.09.005
47. R.A. Doggett, A.M. Krasno, L.K. Koegel, R.L. Koegel, Acquisition of multiple questions in the context of social conversation in children with autism. J. Autism Dev. Disord. **43**(9), 2015–2025 (2013). https://doi.org/10.1007/s10803-012-1749-8
48. L.C. Chezan, E. Drasgow, E.M. Grybos, Conversation skills and self-initiated interactions in young adults with autism and intellectual disability. Res. Autism Spectr. Disord. **75**, 101554 (2020). https://doi.org/10.1016/j.rasd.2020.101554
49. P. Trower, Situational analysis of the components and processes of behavior of socially skilled and unskilled patients. J. Consult. Clin. Psychol. **48**(3), 327–339 (1980). https://doi.org/10.1037/0022-006X.48.3.327
50. P.M. Monti et al., Multi-modal measurement of anxiety and social skills in a behavioral role-play test: Generalizability and discriminant validity. Behav. Assess. **6**(1), 15–25 (1984)
51. G.C. Harb, W. Eng, T. Zaider, R.G. Heimberg, Behavioral assessment of public-speaking anxiety using a modified version of the Social Performance Rating Scale. Behav. Res. Ther. **41**(11), 1373–1380 (2003). https://doi.org/10.1016/S0005-7967(03)00158-X
52. N. Lau, A.M. Zhou, A. Yuan, R. Parigoris, A.R. Rosenberg, J.R. Weisz, Social Skills Deficits and Self-appraisal Biases in Children with Social Anxiety Disorder. J. Child Fam. Stud. (2022). https://doi.org/10.1007/s10826-021-02194-w
53. P. Trower, Skills training for adolescent social problems: a viable treatment alternative? J. Adolesc. **1**(4), 319–329 (1978). https://doi.org/10.1016/S0140-1971(78)80035-9

54. P.E. Shrout, J.L. Fleiss, Intraclass correlations: uses in assessing rater reliability, Psychol. Bull. **86**(2), 420–428 (1979). https://doi.org/10.1037//0033-2909.86.2.420
55. N. Abe, K. Abe, K. Nakashima, The role of perceived stress and fear of negative evaluation in the process from alexithymia to over-adaptation. Psychologia **62**(3–4), 217–232 (2020). https://doi.org/10.2117/psysoc.2020-A001
56. R.M. Bagby, G.J. Taylor, J.D.A. Parker, The twenty-item Toronto alexithymia scale—II. Convergent, discriminant, and concurrent validity. J. Psychosom. Res. **38**(1), 33–40 (1994). https://doi.org/10.1016/0022-3999(94)90006-X
57. R.P. Mattick, J.C. Clarke, Development and validation of measures of social phobia scrutiny fear and social interaction anxiety. Behav. Res. Ther. **36**(4), 455–470 (1998). https://doi.org/10.1016/s0005-7967(97)10031-6
58. J. Delay, P. Pichot, T. Lemperiere, R. Mirouze, La nosologie des états dépressifs. Rapports entre l'etiologie et la sémiologie: II. Résultats du questionnaire de Beck. [The nosology of the depressive states: relations between etiology and semiology: II. results of Beck's questionnaire.]. Encéphale Rev. Psychiatr. Clin. Biol. Thérapeutique **52**(6), 497–504 (1963)
59. A.T. Beck, A. Beamesderfer, Assessment of depression: the depression inventory. Mod. Probl. Pharmacopsychiatry **7**, 151–169 (1974). https://doi.org/10.1159/000395074
60. A. Costello, J. Osborne, Best practices in exploratory factor analysis: four recommendations for getting the most from your analysis, Pract. Assess. Res. Eval. **10**(1), (2019). https://doi.org/10.7275/jyj1-4868
61. A. Beavers, J. Lounsbury, J. Richards, S. Huck, G. Skolits, S. Esquivel, Practical considerations for using exploratory factor analysis in educational research, Pract. Assess. Res. Eval. **18**(1) 2019, https://doi.org/10.7275/qv2q-rk76
62. W.F. Velicer, Determining the number of components from the matrix of partial correlations. Psychometrika **41**(3), 321–327 (1976). https://doi.org/10.1007/BF02293557
63. L.J. Cronbach, Coefficient alpha and the internal structure of tests. Psychometrika **16**(3), 297–334 (1951). https://doi.org/10.1007/BF02310555
64. T.K. Koo, M.Y. Li, A Guideline of Selecting and Reporting Intraclass Correlation Coefficients for Reliability Research. J. Chiropr. Med. **15**(2), 155–163 (2016). https://doi.org/10.1016/j.jcm.2016.02.012
65. K.A. Smith-Jentsch, J.H. Johnston, S.C. Payne, Measuring team-related expertise in complex environments, in *Making decisions under stress: Implications for individual and team training*, (Washington, DC, US: American Psychological Association, 1998), pp. 61–87. https://doi.org/10.1037/10278-003
66. M. Dindar, S. Järvelä, H. Järvenoja, Interplay of metacognitive experiences and performance in collaborative problem solving. Comput. Educ. **154**, 103922 (2020). https://doi.org/10.1016/j.compedu.2020.103922

Eye-Gaze Analysis

Kana Miyamoto and Kosuke Okazaki

Abstract This chapter explains eye movements during collaborative problem-solving. Collaborative problem-solving means resolving difficulties and working toward a goal during social collaboration with others. Social life is filled with collaborative problem-solving tasks, such as group work in schools or workplaces. Understanding behavioral signals is one important step in improving performance in collaborative problem-solving. We focus on eye movements as an example in this section. We show the analyses of eye movements related to social performance and discuss future directions for investigating eye movements to improve collaborative problem-solving.

1 Introduction

1.1 Collaborative Problem-Solving

Collaborative problem-solving is a process in which a group works together to address a common problem [1]. Collaborative problem-solving tasks include group work at school and project activities for work. In recent years, collaborative problem-solving skills have gained attention as an important twenty-first-century skill [2]. Such skills are associated with both social and cognitive skills [3–5]. The former is comprised of the collaborative part of collaborative problem-solving. The ability to successfully use social skills in social situations is referred to as social performance. A dysfunction of social performance might lead to experiencing negative situations [6], for example, conflicts with people and feelings of loneliness or anxiety. These negative aspects cause difficulties in interpersonal relationships and

K. Miyamoto (✉)
NTT, Musashino, Japan
e-mail: kana.miyamoto@ntt.com

K. Okazaki
Children's Mental Health Center, Shigisan Hospital, Ikoma, Japan
e-mail: okazaki-k@heartland.or.jp

S. Nakamura (ed.), *Multimodal Interaction Technologies for Training Affective Social Skills*, https://doi.org/10.1007/978-981-96-1313-7_6

reduce one's quality of life. High social performance molds appropriate behaviors in a variety of social situations and builds good relationships with others. Understanding and enhancing social performance is critical in practical situations, including collaborative problem-solving.

A social performance rating scale (SPRS), which is one evaluation method of social performance [7], consists of five items: gaze, voice quality, length, discomfort, and conversation flow. These items are evaluated on a five-point Likert scale from 1 to 5. The SPRS is a validated scale developed in English [7], French [8], and Japanese [9]. Its English version was applied to videos of a simulated dinner party for three cohorts of participants: those with a primary diagnosis of social phobia, those with a primary diagnosis of an anxiety disorder, and control participants. The French version was applied to videos of collaborative games for neurotypical participants. The Japanese version was applied to videos of social skill training for controls, autism spectrum disorder, and schizophrenia. The SPRS is available in several languages and is often used in a variety of research to measure social performance [10].

A SPRS measurement during a collaborative problem-solving task provides an evaluation of the social domain of collaborative problem-solving skills. Although the SPRS can be measured from the description of the above five items, the detailed characteristics of behavioral signals are unclear for obtaining a high SPRS. For example, the highest score of the gaze item is defined as "participant keeps eye contact during the conversation, does not stare, and shifts focus during pauses and conversation [7]". It is uncertain what length of gaze time is associated with a higher SPRS. Previous studies have focused on social performance and individual characteristics or on individual characteristics and behavioral signals. We conjectured that perhaps looking for the characteristics of behavioral signals associated with social performance might provide clues for improving it. Therefore, we investigated the relationship between such behavioral signals as eye movements and social performance during a collaborative problem-solving task.

1.2 Individual Characteristics and Social Performance

Several studies indicated that individual characteristics are associated with social performance [6]. For example, people with high anxiety tendencies during social interactions attempt to conceal such manifestations of anxiety as blushing, trembling, and sweating [11]. They more often subjectively evaluate their own social performance as lower than healthy people [12]. Some studies report that in objective evaluations, people with high anxiety tendencies also have deficits in social performance [13], although other studies report no difference in the social performance between people with high anxiety tendencies and the healthy [14]. Alexithymia, another individual characteristic that affects social performance, is characterized by the difficulty of recognizing and verbally expressing emotions as well as a lack of fantasy and imagination. These symptoms impair important functions in social interaction and affect social communication [15]. Reports have also described significant differences in SPRS evaluations with high alexithymia tendencies [16]. According to previous studies, such individual characteristics as anxiety and alexithymia may influence social performance.

1.3 Eye Movements and Social Performance

Eye movements, which are crucial components for expressing one's message to others, are related to social performance [17]. SPRS contains a gaze item. In it, the lowest score is defined as "participant completely avoids looking at the partner or stares continually." Avoiding eye contact indicates anxiety or discomfort in social interaction. On the other hand, an excessively long gaze is not acceptable, either. A speaker commonly gazes at a listener who looks around the speaker's face. Eye movements are also affected by turn-taking. When a speaker wants to continue talking, he removes his gaze, and when a listener wants to start speaking, she shifts her gaze to the speaker. Eye movements contain various meanings in social communication [18].

Eye movements are also influenced by individual characteristics. Previous studies have shown that people with anxiety tend to avoid eye contact [19, 20]. Reduced eye contact has been reported, especially when a person confronts an angry expression [21]. Similar results where people avoid looking at a face have been identified in people with alexithymia [22]. People with anxiety or alexithymia tend to avoid looking at other people's faces.

1.4 Social Performance and Eye Movements During Collaborative Problem-Solving Tasks

We introduce previous studies that have focused on collaborative problem-solving tasks. Hamet Bagnou et al. [8] investigated the relationship between social performance during collaborative problem-solving and tendencies to experience anxiety and alexithymia. The study recorded two participants talking through an online communication tool. The annotators evaluated the participants' social performances using SPRS [7] and found that participants with a high tendency toward anxiety have low SPRS scores.

Other studies investigated eye movements during collaborative problem-solving tasks. Celepkolu and Boyer [23] investigated eye movements while two participants were doing collaborative programming. Their results showed that the participants' eye movements can provide predictive insight into their post-test scores. Macdonald and Tatler [24] investigated eye movements while two participants baked together and concluded that social context can affect the behavioral signals of eye movements during social interaction.

Andrist, Ruis, and Shaffer [25] used epistemic network analysis to model the eye movements while two participants were working on a sandwich-building task. As described above, eye movements have been explored during collaborative problem-solving tasks. However, relatively little attention has focused on eye movements and social performance. We believe that identifying eye movements related to social performance during such tasks will improve social performance.

We introduce the dataset for analysis of eye movements and social performance in Sect. 2 and show details of the analyses in Sect. 3. Finally, we summarize the analyses of eye movements and discuss future directions in Sect. 4.

2 Japanese Version of TALENT Dataset

We present a Japanese version TALENT dataset for analyses of eye movements and social performance during a collaborative problem-solving task. Hamet Bagnou et al. [8] created a collaboraTive sociAL skills and attenTion (TALENT) dataset which includes profiles and recordings while two participants engage in collaborative problem-solving tasks online. We followed the data recording procedures of their TALENT dataset and created the Japanese version.

2.1 Participants

Fifty healthy participants took part in the data collection (age: 39.4 ± 11.0 years old; 25 males, 25 females). We set up pairs of participants to work on a cooperative problem-solving task via an online communication tool. We recorded their activities on the task and collected questionnaires about anxiety and alexithymia. This data collection was approved by the Research Ethics Committee of the Nara Institute of Science and Technology (Approval No. 2022-I-60).

2.2 Recording of Behavioral Signals

We show the method for measuring the participants' behaviors. A small room with a chair and a desk was prepared for each of the two participants, and their behaviors during a collaborative problem-solving task were measured. Three laptop computers for the two participants and an experimenter were prepared and connected via BigBlueButton, which is an online communication tool. Participants wore headphones and worked on the task through the BigBlueButton. The two participants' activities were observed with headphones and webcams installed on the top of the laptop monitor. We set up the BigBlueButton so that the two participants viewed side-by-side on the monitor. The BigBlueButton screen and audio of the participants were recorded by Open Broadcaster Software using the experimenter's laptop. In addition, eye movements were measured with an eye tracker (Tobii Pro Fusion) attached to the lower part of the participant's laptop monitor. The sampling rate was 30 Hz, with a resolution of 192 × 1080. Before the measurements, we calibrated the eye tracker using Tobii Pro Lab.

2.3 *Questionnaire*

We collected three types of questionnaires. For measurement of anxiety, we used two questionnaires: a Japanese version of Social Interaction Anxiety Scale (SIAS) [26] and a Japanese version of State-Trait Anxiety Inventory (STAI) [27]. The SIAS measures anxiety about social interactions. The scale is composed of 20 items, and the items are scored ranging from 0 to 4. The STAI measures general anxiety and consists of a state anxiety scale (STAI-state) and a trait anxiety scale (STAI-trait). Both scales have 20 items. The items are scored ranging from 1 to 4. We used an alexithymia questionnaire: a Japanese version of The 20-item Toronto Alexithymia Scale (TAS-20) [28]. It consists of 20 items and measures three scales: difficulty identifying feelings (DIF), difficulty describing feelings (DDF), and externally oriented thinking (EOT). The items are scored ranging from 1 to 5. We calculated the total score of the three scales. The scores of the anxiety and alexithymia questionnaires for the 50 participants in this data collection are shown in Table 1.

We show the recording procedure. First, the two participants and the experimenter each entered a separate room. We explained the data recording process to the participants and gave them instructions mainly via the online communication tool BigBlueButton. The participants took an explanation of the data recording and filled out a consent form. They then completed three questionnaires: the SIAS and STAI for anxiety, and the TAS-20 for alexithymia. Next, we provided information about the collaborative problem-solving task. In this study, we conducted a task in which two participants cooperated in a discussion about survival. The task was to discuss items necessary for survival, assuming a situation in which a plane crash-landed on a mountain [8, 29]. Since this task is performed orally, no tools, such as a whiteboard, are needed. It is expected to promote natural interaction. The time limit was five

Table 1 Questionnaire scores for anxiety and alexithymia in our data collection

	SIAS	STAI-state	STAI-trait	TAS-20
Average	28.2	42.0	46.2	44.8
SD	11.7	8.89	10.5	11.3
Min	12	22	25	23
Max	56	59	71	74

Table 2 Inter-rater reliability for the SPRS during collaborative problem-solving

Item	ICC 2 K
Gaze	0.789
Voice quality	0.851
Length	0.761
Discomfort	0.832
Conversation flow	0.823

minutes, and participants' behavior while working on the task was measured using headsets, webcams, and eye tracker devices.

2.4 Annotation of Social Performance

We annotated the participants' social performances during the collaborative problem-solving task using a SPRS [7]. In our study, three third-party raters evaluated the social performance by its Japanese version. The raters watched five videos and discussed the SPRS content for evaluation practice and then evaluated the scores of the other videos without any discussion. They were not told anything about the scores of the questionnaires concerning anxiety and alexithymia. We measured the inter-rater agreement by calculating the intraclass correlation coefficient (ICC, 2 k) for the validation of the SPRS annotated by the three raters. We opted for the random two-way ICC method with the mean as the unit of evaluation shown in Table 2. The intraclass correlation coefficients ranged from 0 to 1, and all items had reliability values between 0.761 and 0.851. The intraclass correlation coefficients were above 0.75, which indicates good reliability [30]. The score for each SPRS item was averaged for the three raters' annotations in subsequent analyses. We used total scores of the SPRS items for the analyses.

2.5 Preprocessing

We used Tobii Pro Lab to preprocess the eye movements recorded during the collaborative problem-solving task. Three areas of interest (AOI) were set up to determine where participants looked during the task shown in Fig. 1: The first AOI was the area on the left side of the screen where participants looked at themselves (self); the second AOI was the area on the right side of the screen where participants looked at their conversation partners (other); and the third AOI was the area on online communication tools other than self and other or the area outside the screen (outside).

We computed the features based on eye movements to look at a specific position, called fixation. Fixations are detected every time frame in the Tobii Pro Lab. We

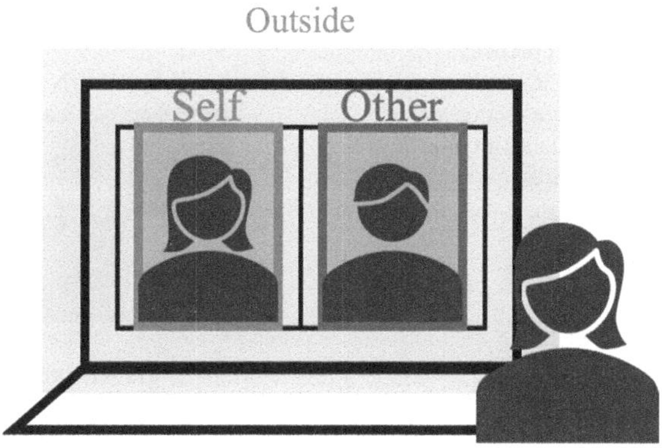

Fig. 1 Areas of interest for eye movements analysis

calculated the total time of fixations detected at each AOI. However, frames may contain errors, such as eyes not being detected, and the number of frames available for feature extraction varies from participant to participant. Therefore, we calculated the proportion of the time of fixation in the self, other, and outside areas. In other words, we calculated features that express the percentage of looking at the self, other, and outside areas; the sum of the percentage of looking at the three AOIs is 1.

We also calculated features separately for whether the participants were speaking or listening. A previous study provides the reference that people with social anxiety do not look at their conversation partners when they are listening to them, compared to people without social anxiety [20, 31]. Therefore, we conducted an analysis that took into account the participants' speech state. First, we used Speaker Diarization Using OpenAI Whisper [32] to detect speech segments. Then, we calculated the percentage of participants looking at each of the three areas when they were speaking and when they were listening to their partner.

3 Analysis of Eye Movements

3.1 Analysis of Social Performance and Individual Characteristics

Previous studies showed correlations between trends in social performance and individual characteristics. We first examined if the same results will be found in our dataset. We have one hypothesis: participants with high tendencies of anxiety or alexithymia have low SPRS scores. To test the hypothesis, we used Spearman's rank correlation coefficients between SPRS and questionnaire scores.

The correlation coefficients between SPRS and questionnaire scores are shown in Fig. 2. The SPRS score was negatively correlated with SIAS ($p = 0.01$), STAI ($p <$

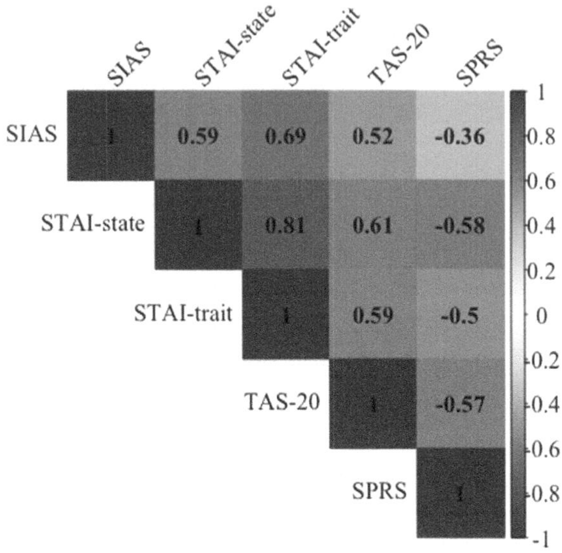

Fig. 2 Spearman's rank correlation coefficient between SPRS and questionnaires scores of anxiety and alexithymia questionnaires

0.001), and TAS-20 ($p < 0.001$). In addition, there were positive correlations among the questionnaires for anxiety and alexithymia.

We tested Spearman's rank correlation coefficient SPRS and questionnaire scores. We found negative correlations between SPRS and SIAS, STAI, or TAS-20. This supports the hypothesis that participants with high tendencies of anxiety or alexithymia have low SPRS scores. Thus, we showed the same results as the previous study that investigated social performance and individual characteristics during collaborative problem-solving tasks [8].

We also found significant positive correlations among questionnaires of anxiety and alexithymia. Previous studies have shown that anxiety and alexithymia are related, and we consider that our results show the same [33, 34].

3.2 *Analysis of Eye Movements and Individual Characteristics*

We investigated whether individual characteristics impact eye movements. We have two hypotheses: participants with high anxiety tendencies look at their conversation partners less, and participants with high alexithymia tendencies look at their conversation partners less. To test the two hypotheses, we conducted a correlation analysis between eye movements and anxiety and alexithymia tendencies. Spearman's rank correlation coefficients were used for questionnaires regarding anxiety and alexithymia and the percentage of looking at self, other, and outside.

We show Spearman's rank correlation coefficients in Table 3. First, we show the analysis using the overall eye movement data regardless of the participants' speech segments. The percentage of looking at the self area was not significantly correlated with the anxiety and alexithymia questionnaires. The percentage of looking at the other area was negatively correlated with the STAI-state ($\rho = -0.314$, $p = 0.026$), STAI-trait ($\rho = -0.456$, $p < 0.001$), and TAS-20 ($\rho = -0.403$, $p = 0.004$). The percentage of looking at the outside area was positively correlated with STAI-state ($\rho = 0.303$, $p = 0.033$) and STAI-trait ($\rho = 0.336$, $p = 0.017$). These results indicate that the higher the STAI score, the lower the percentage of looking at the conversation partner, and the higher the percentage of looking outside. In addition, higher scores on the TAS-20 were associated with lower percentages of looking at the conversation partner. However, among the anxieties, the SIAS on social interaction was not significantly correlated with the percentage of looking at any of the three AOIs.

Next, we analyzed the eye movement data considering the participants' speech segments. We report on the analysis when participants were speaking first. The percentage of looking at the self area was not significantly correlated with the anxiety and alexithymia questionnaires. The percentage of looking at the other area was negatively correlated with the STAI state ($\rho = -0.335$, $p = 0.017$), STAI trait ($\rho = -0.445$, $p = 0.001$), and TAS-20 ($\rho = -0.383$, $p = 0.006$). The percentage of looking at the outside area was positively correlated with STAI state ($\rho = 0.309$, $p = 0.029$) and STAI trait ($\rho = 0.308$, $p = 0.030$). Then, we report on the analysis when participants were listening. The percentage of looking at the self area was not significantly correlated with the anxiety and alexithymia questionnaires. The percentage of looking at the other area was negatively correlated with the SIAS ($\rho = -0.320$, $p = 0.023$), STAI trait ($\rho = -0.373$, $p = 0.008$), and TAS-20 ($\rho = -0.382$, $p = 0.006$). There was a marginally significant percentage of looking at the other area and STAI state ($\rho = -0.272$, $p = 0.056$). The percentage of looking at the outside area was positively correlated with SIAS ($\rho = 0.337$, $p = 0.017$), STAI state ($\rho = 0.303$, $p = 0.032$), and STAI trait ($\rho = 0.317$, $p = 0.025$). In contrast to the analysis using data from the whole conversation and data while speaking, there were significant correlations between other and SIAS and between outside and SIAS by using data while listening.

We tested Spearman's rank correlation coefficient on the eye movements and questionnaires of anxiety and alexithymia. We found a negative correlation between the percentage of looking at the conversational partner and the STAI score. This supports hypothesis 1 that people with a high anxiety tendency have a low percentage of looking at their conversation partners. We also found a negative correlation between the percentage of looking at the conversation partner and the TAS-20 score. This supports Hypothesis 2 that people with a high alexithymia tendency have a low percentage of looking at the conversation partner. Therefore, we confirmed that the same results as in the previous studies [20, 22] on which the hypothesis was based can be obtained during an online collaborative problem-solving task. In addition, there was a positive correlation between the percentage of looking outside and STAI scores. This result suggests that people with high anxiety tendencies avoid looking at other people's faces regardless of whether those faces are their own or those of

Table 3 Spearman's correlation between eye movements and questionnaire scores (*$p < 0.05$, **$p < 0.01$, ***$p < 0.001$)

		AOI of all data			AOI for speaking data			AOI for listening data		
		Self	Other	Outside	Self	Other	Outside	Self	Other	Outside
SIAS	ρ	− 0.069	− 0.232	0.222	− 0.111	− 0.208	0.147	− 0.030	− 0.320*	0.337*
	p	0.633	0.105	0.121	0.442	0.148	0.307	0.836	0.023	0.017
STAI-state	ρ	− 0.004	− 0.314*	0.303*	0.002	− 0.335*	0.309*	0.001	− 0.272	0.303*
	p	0.980	0.026	0.033	0.987	0.017	0.029	0.993	0.056	0.032
STAI-trait	ρ	0.144	− 0.456***	0.336*	0.143	− 0.445**	0.308*	0.124	− 0.373**	0.317*
	p	0.317	< 0.001	0.017	0.321	0.001	0.030	0.392	0.008	0.025
TAS-20	ρ	0.213	− 0.403**	0.220	0.196	− 0.383**	0.218	0.225	− 0.382**	0.257
	p	0.138	0.004	0.125	0.172	0.006	0.129	0.117	0.006	0.072

Fig. 3 Percentage looking outside while speaking and listening

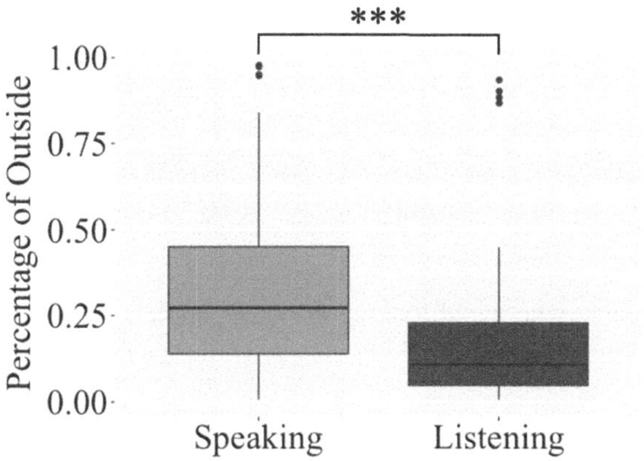

their conversation partners. There was a significant correlation between SIAS and the percentage of looking at the conversation partner or outside only during listening. This result is consistent with the results of the previous study [20]. Figure 3 is boxplots showing the percentage of participants looking outside while speaking and listening. We used Wilcoxon sign-rank test, and the results showed that a greater proportion of participants looked outside while speaking than while listening. We consider that many participants looked well outside while speaking, and there was no difference in eye movements between those with social anxiety and those without.

3.3 Analysis of Eye Movements and Social Performance

Finally, we investigated our main topic which is the relationship between eye movements and social performance. We have one hypothesis: participants who look at their conversation partners less have low SPRS scores. This hypothesis was set out from two previous analyses. To test the hypothesis, we used Spearman's rank correlation coefficients between eye movements and SPRS.

The correlation coefficients between eye movements and SPRS score are shown in Table 4. The percentage of looking at the other area was positively correlated with SPRS score, even when using eye movement features using all data, speaking data, and listening data. The percentage of looking at the outside area was negatively correlated with the SPRS score when using eye movement features using all data and listening data.

We tested Spearman's rank correlation coefficient on eye movements and SPRS. We found a positive correlation between the percentage of looking at the conversational partner and SPRS. This supports the hypothesis that participants who look at their conversation partners less have low SPRS scores. In addition, there was a negative correlation between the percentage of looking outside and SPRS, except when using eye movement features using speaking data. This result suggests that

Table 4 Spearman's correlation between eye movements and the total of SPRS items (* $p < 0.05$, ** $p < 0.01$, *** $p < 0.001$)

		AOI of all data			AOI for speaking data			AOI for listening data		
		Self	Other	Outside	Self	Other	Outside	Self	Other	Outside
SIAS	ρ	− 0.259	0.547***	− 0.339*	− 0.215	0.486**	− 0.251	− 0.268	0.541***	− 0.456***
	p	0.069	<0.001	0.016	0.133	<0.001	0.079	0.060	<0.001	<0.001

people who avoid looking at other people's faces were evaluated with low SPRS scores. However, looking outside while speaking may not affect the SPRS score.

4 Summary and Future Direction

We collected data during collaborative problem-solving tasks online and conducted three types of analyses: social performance and individual characteristics, eye movements and individual characteristics, and eye movements and social performance. We showed that anxiety and alexithymia are related to social performance. These tendencies influence eye movements. Furthermore, eye movements are related to social performance, suggesting that looking at a conversation partner and avoiding looking outside might be one solution for improving social performance. In our analyses, we set three AOIs: self, other, and outside. Assuming face-to-face conversations, we might need to include the self area in the outside area. Perhaps we will further consider AOIs in the future. We also did not consider the effects of eye movement due to turn-taking. Previous studies showed that speakers look away at the beginning of speech and turn their gaze toward the listener when they finish speaking [35]. Analysis that takes into account turn-taking effects is our future work.

The limitation of this work is that the data were analyzed using only Japanese people. Differences in eye movements exist between the Western and Eastern worlds [36]. Therefore, the values for the percentage of looking at AOI in our experiment may differ between countries. However, we showed significant correlations between eye movements and individual characteristics and social performance, similar to the results shown in previous studies that did not use Japanese data. Thus, although perhaps country-specific and culture-specific differences might be found in the characteristics of eye movements, we believe that the relationship between them and individual characteristics and social performance is broadly the same.

Acknowledgements This chapter is mainly modified from the PhD thesis of the first author and extended for this publication. Funding was provided by the Core Research for Evolutionary Science and Technology (Grant No. JPMJCR19A5). The chapter's contents are excerpted from an article currently under review at Acta Psychologica: https://papers.ssrn.com/sol3/papers.cfm?abstract_id=4889867.

References

1. A.K. Ahonen, S.M. Harding, Assessing online collaborative problem solving among school children in Finland: a case study using ATC21S TM in a national context. Int. J. Learn. Teach. Educ. Res. **17**(2), 138–158 (2018). https://doi.org/10.26803/ijlter.17.2.9
2. OECD, *PISA 2015 Assessment and Analytical Framework: Science, Reading, Mathematic, Financial Literacy and Collaborative Problem Solving*. Paris: Organisation for Economic Co-operation and Development, 2017. Accessed: Aug. 23, 2024. [Online]. Available: https://www.oecd-ilibrary.org/education/pisa-2015-assessment-and-analytical-framework_9789264281820-en
3. F. Hesse, E. Care, J. Buder, K. Sassenberg, P. Griffin, A Framework for Teachable Collaborative Problem Solving Skills, in *Assessment and Teaching of 21st Century Skills*, P. Griffin and E. Care, Eds., Dordrecht: Springer Netherlands, pp. 37–56. (2015) https://doi.org/10.1007/978-94-017-9395-7_2
4. C. Scoular, E. Care, Monitoring patterns of social and cognitive student behaviors in online collaborative problem solving assessments. Comput. Hum. Behav. **104**, 105874 (2020)
5. C. Sun et al., The relationship between collaborative problem solving behaviors and solution outcomes in a game-based learning environment. Comput. Hum. Behav. **128**, 107120 (2022)
6. S. Marwaha, S. Johnson, Schizophrenia and employment. Soc. Psychiatry Psychiatr. Epidemiol. **39**(5), 337–349 (2004). https://doi.org/10.1007/s00127-004-0762-4
7. T. Fydrich, D.L. Chambless, K.J. Perry, F. Buergener, M.B. Beazley, Behavioral assessment of social performance: a rating system for social phobia. Behav. Res. Ther. **36**(10), 995–1010 (1998). https://doi.org/10.1016/S0005-7967(98)00069-2
8. J. Hamet Bagnou, E. Prigent, J.C. Martin, C. Clavel, Adaptation and validation of two annotation scales for assessing social skills in a corpus of multimodal collaborative interactions. Front. Psychol. **27**(13), 1039169 (2022). https://doi.org/10.3389/fpsyg.2022.1039169
9. K. Miyamoto *et al.*, Social performance rating during social skills training in adults with autism spectrum disorder and schizophrenia, in *2023 11th International Conference on Affective Computing and Intelligent Interaction Workshops and Demos (ACIIW)*, IEEE, pp. 1–8. (2023) Accessed: Aug. 23, 2024. [Online]. Available: https://ieeexplore.ieee.org/abstract/document/10388083/
10. S. Stevens, R. Cooper, T. Bantin, C. Hermann, A.L. Gerlach, Feeling safe but appearing anxious: differential effects of alcohol on anxiety and social performance in individuals with social anxiety disorder. Behav. Res. Ther. **94**, 9–18 (2017)
11. D.M. Clark, W.R. Crozier, L.E. Alden, A cognitive perspective on social phobia. Essent. Handb. Soc. Anxiety Clin. **4**, 193–218 (2005)
12. J. Asbrand, B. Tuschen-Caffier, Taking a closer look at social performance in childhood social anxiety disorder: biopsychosocial context considerations and effects of cognitive behavior therapy. Children **9**(10), 1515 (2022). https://doi.org/10.3390/children9101515
13. M.J. Voncken, S.M. Bögels, Social performance deficits in social anxiety disorder: reality during conversation and biased perception during speech. J. Anxiety Disord. **22**(8), 1384–1392 (2008). https://doi.org/10.1016/j.janxdis.2008.02.001
14. T. Thompson, N. Van Zalk, C. Marshall, M. Sargeant, B. Stubbs, Social anxiety increases visible anxiety signs during social encounters but does not impair performance. BMC Psychol. **7**(1), 1–9 (2019). https://doi.org/10.1186/s40359-019-0300-5
15. E.B. Dalokay, A. Aydin, The relationship between alexithymia, communication skills and mental well-being of nurses' in Turkey: a cross-sectional study. Arch. Psychiatr. Nurs. **1**(43), 81–86 (2023). https://doi.org/10.1016/j.apnu.2022.12.020
16. O. Pollatos et al., Differential effects of alexithymia subscales on autonomic reactivity and anxiety during social stress. J. Psychosom. Res. **70**(6), 525–533 (2011). https://doi.org/10.1016/j.jpsychores.2010.12.003
17. A.S. Bellack, K.T. Mueser, S. Gingerich, J. Agresta, *Social Skills Training for Schizophrenia: A Step-by-Step Guide*. Guilford Publications, (2013)

18. A. Kendon, Some functions of gaze-direction in social interaction. Acta Psychol. Amst **26**, 22–63 (1967)
19. K. Horley, L.M. Williams, C. Gonsalvez, E. Gordon, Face to face: visual scanpath evidence for abnormal processing of facial expressions in social phobia. Psychiatry Res. **127**(1–2), 43–53 (2004)
20. J. Chen, E. Van Den Bos, J.D. Karch, P.M. Westenberg, Social anxiety is related to reduced face gaze during a naturalistic social interaction. Anxiety Stress Coping **36**(4), 460–474 (2023). https://doi.org/10.1080/10615806.2022.2125961
21. L.F. Van Dillen, D. Enter, L.P. Peters, W.W. van Dijk, M. Rotteveel, Moral fixations: the role of moral integrity and social anxiety in the selective avoidance of social threat. Biol. Psychol. **122**, 51–58 (2017)
22. G. Bird, C. Press, D.C. Richardson, The role of alexithymia in reduced eye-fixation in autism spectrum conditions. J. Autism Dev. Disord. **41**(11), 1556–1564 (2011). https://doi.org/10.1007/s10803-011-1183-3
23. M. Celepkolu, K.E. Boyer, *Predicting Student Performance Based on Eye Gaze During Collaborative Problem Solving* (Group Interaction Frontiers in Technology. GIFT, Proc, 2018). https://doi.org/10.1145/3279981.3279991
24. R.G. Macdonald, B.W. Tatler, Gaze in a real-world social interaction: a dual eye-tracking study. Q. J. Exp. Psychol. **71**(10), 2162–2173 (2018). https://doi.org/10.1177/1747021817739221
25. S. Andrist, A.R. Ruis, D.W. Shaffer, A network analytic approach to gaze coordination during a collaborative task. Comput. Hum. Behav. **89**, 339–348 (2018)
26. Y. Kanai, Development and validation of the Japanese version of social phobia scale and social interaction anxiety scale. Jpn. J. Psychosom. Med. **44**, 841 (2004)
27. T. Hidano, M. Fukuhara, S. Iwawaki, C.D.S. Soga, *State-Trait Anxiety Inventory-JYZ* (Practical Education Publishing, Tokyo, 2000)
28. K. Gen et al., The reliability and factorial validity of the Japanese version of the 20-item Toronto alexithymia scale (TAS-20). Jpn. J. Psychosom. Med. **43**, 839–846 (2003)
29. J. Hall, W.H. Watson, The effects of a normative intervention on group decision-making performance. Hum. Relat. **23**(4), 299–317 (1970)
30. T.K. Koo, M.Y. Li, A guideline of selecting and reporting intraclass correlation coefficients for reliability research. J. Chiropr. Med. **15**(2), 155–163 (2016)
31. J. Chen, E. van den Bos, S. L.M. Velthuizen, P.M. Westenberg, Visual avoidance of faces in socially anxious individuals: the moderating effect of type of social situation, *J. Exp. Psychopathol.*, vol. 12, no. 1, (2021), https://doi.org/10.1177/2043808721989628
32. M. Ashraf, *Speaker Diarization Using OpenAI Whisper*. (2023). [Online]. Available: https://github.com/MahmoudAshraf97/whisper-diarization#speaker-diarization-using-openai-whisper
33. D. Berardis et al., The impact of alexithymia on anxiety disorders: a review of the literature. Curr. Psychiatry Rev. **4**(2), 80–86 (2008). https://doi.org/10.2174/157340008784529287
34. M. Karukivi et al., Alexithymia is associated with anxiety among adolescents. J. Affect. Disord. **125**(1–3), 383–387 (2010). https://doi.org/10.1016/j.jad.2010.02.126
35. R. Cañigueral, A.F. Hamilton, The role of eye gaze during natural social interactions in typical and autistic people. Front. Psychol. **10**, 1–18 (2019). https://doi.org/10.3389/fpsyg.2019.00560
36. J.X. Haensel, T.J. Smith, A. Senju, Cultural differences in mutual gaze during face-to-face interactions: a dual head-mounted eye-tracking study. Vis. Cogn. **30**(1–2), 100–115 (2022). https://doi.org/10.1080/13506285.2021.1928354

Multimodal Behavior Modeling

Takeshi Saga and Hiroki Tanaka

Abstract This chapter explains the complexities of multimodal behavior modeling. While humans recognize social intentions unconsciously, the automation of such recognition involves significant challenges, particularly in spontaneous interactions. We explore the variety of multimodal behavior modeling through two specific examples—ASD severity estimation and social skill estimation—to showcase its potential. Using datasets from clinical populations and machine learning techniques, the chapter demonstrates the potential analytic power of automatic behavior modeling with multimodal features like text, audio, and visual cues. We also discuss expected challenges in this field in the era of LLMs, such as the need for sequential modeling and the limited amount of data. Accordingly, we hope to show the future direction of multimodal behavior modeling.

1 Introduction

Social communication is the process of sharing ideas, beliefs, and values among groups through various forms of communication, such as spoken and written words, images, and gestures [1]. Although we recognize the social intentions of interlocutors unconsciously, the automatic measurement of intentions is challenging in general. To understand a person's intentions from the above information sources, it is necessary to appropriately integrate multimodal behavior signals and analyze them. Although human beings can easily evaluate these multimodal communicative signals, their computational analysis needs sophisticated techniques. In particular, automatic measurement in spontaneous settings is technically challenging. In this chapter, we showcase what we can do with the current technologies and introduce the challenges we still need to overcome.

T. Saga (✉)
ISIR, Sorbonne University, Paris, France
e-mail: takeshi.saga@isir.upmc.fr

H. Tanaka
International Christian University, Mitaka, Japan
e-mail: hiroki.tanaka@icu.ac.jp

S. Nakamura (ed.), *Multimodal Interaction Technologies for Training Affective Social Skills*, https://doi.org/10.1007/978-981-96-1313-7_7

We first clarify the definition of behavior modeling as used in this chapter and its challenges in computational approaches. Then, we move on to evaluations by human annotators. After that, we introduce actual examples we've investigated and conclude with future prospects of multimodal behavior modeling.

2 Behavior Modeling

In this chapter, we refer to the term "behavior modeling" as the measurement of human communicative behaviors. It is also called "behavior analysis" or simply "measurement of human behaviors." It should be noted that "behavior modeling" in this chapter is a more generic concept than the one used in social skills training (SST) theories. Since humans use not only a signal but multiple signals for communications, we focus on multimodal interactions of human behaviors, including text, audio, face, and body signals.

In contrast, for the following reasons, multimodal signals cannot be easily handled with automatic behavior modeling.

First, there are few shared datasets on communicative interactions [2]. To acquire multimodal data, we need to use a microphone and a video camera for each person. Here, careful attention should be given to microphone selection to prevent a person's voice from being captured by the interlocutor's microphone, which makes it very difficult to analyze the audio interaction between them. Therefore, we need to use a microphone that captures only close sounds, and thus one for professional musical use or for live streaming would be a great choice. Additional devices, such as a depth camera or a heart-rate monitor might be needed depending on the purpose. If it is a two-person interaction, two sets of these devices are required, which is time- and cost-intensive. Furthermore, we also need to consider privacy concerns if we intend to make results open to the public. Since we need to overcome all of these issues when creating a dataset of reasonable quality, there are few publicly available high-quality datasets on multimodal interactions.

Second, even when public datasets are available, they often have quality issues [2]. For example, they cannot be used when there is too much noise or missing data about the conversation partner. Furthermore, when the dataset is small, there are fewer methods available for analysis, and we cannot use powerful deep neural networks.

Third, interactions among multiple signals are complicated [3]. Since social signals act in a complementary manner, all signals must be treated simultaneously as time-series signals. Since we don't have much data, we need to synchronize and find interactions in detail without using neural network training, which is still a challenging task to solve.

Fourth, social signals can be ambiguous [4]. In addition to multiple interpretations depending on the surrounding context, sometimes, there might be multiple possible candidates for the specific context. Human beings usually infer which intention is correct or directly ask the interlocutor for the actual intentions. However, when and how to take those strategies automatically is another difficult challenge.

Considering these challenges in multimodal behavior modeling, we pursued strategies to collect our own small-sized dataset under interaction conditions that are as natural as possible. Moreover, we used conventional but robust machine-learning models to solve each of our problems. In this chapter, we elaborate on two example cases: multimodal ASD severity estimation and social skill estimation.

3 Human Evaluation in Social Interaction

When we communicate with others, we implicitly and unconsciously estimate behaviors subjectively. In contrast, the qualitative or quantitative evaluation of behaviors is still challenging. For instance, in evaluating concrete tasks such as job interviews or situations requiring persuasion, researchers sometimes measure them by task success rate or hireability scores by recruiters. However, unlike those task-oriented behavior measures, general-purpose measures are not common due to the need to cover many aspects of social behaviors.

One example is the revised version of the Japanese role-play test, which is a well-validated evaluation method for social skills that uses a seven-item evaluation metric along with provided social situations [5]. It is composed of seven evaluation items: eye contact, body direction/distance, facial expression, voice variation, clarity, fluency, and social appropriateness to each task. The social appropriateness item is used to cover task-specific necessary skills for each situation, so it differs depending on the SST task. Out of many possible social situations, we chose the four basic social skills defined by Bellack: listening to others (LISTEN), conveying positive feelings (TELL), making a request to others (ASK), and declining a request (DECLINE) [6]. For the LISTEN task, social appropriateness determines whether the participants paid attention to the interlocutor, including nodding, back-channels, and empathetic behaviors. For the TELL task, social appropriateness is about expressing attention to the interlocutor's responses and the suitability of their speech contents. For the ASK task, social appropriateness assesses whether they explained the details of their request, including what kind of help they need. It also includes whether they listened to the interlocutor. For the DECLINE task, social appropriateness involves whether they expressed contriteness and appropriate reasons for a refusal. It also includes whether they proposed alternatives for the request, which is an essential act for the situation. These evaluations are done on a 5-point Likert scale, from 1 (worst) to 5 (best). For instance, the evaluators give 5 points for eye contact if the user's eye contact is natural and occurs with appropriate frequency. Conversely, the evaluators give 1 point if there is no eye contact, potentially causing the interlocutor to feel uncomfortable.

As explained so far, by using well-designed metrics with the help of experienced professional workers, these methods can evaluate social skills by eliminating subjectivity as much as possible. However, this requires a deep understanding of behavioral analyses and undocumented common sense based on years of clinical experience, which makes it difficult to scale up the research or industrial activities. Therefore, methods of automatic evaluation are in demand, and some researchers have already achieved this with the power of machine learning techniques.

4 Examples of Behavior Modeling

In this section, we explain some examples of actual automatic behavior modeling. We used datasets of clinical populations, specifically sufferers of schizophrenia (SZ) and autism spectrum disorder (ASD), for this series of research because these people typically face difficulties in social interactions. Here, automatic behavior modeling can be used to analyze these disorders' mechanisms or to develop assistive applications for improvements.

4.1 Multimodal ASD Severity Estimation

ASD is one of the developmental disorders that causes difficulties in social interactions. People with ASD have problems not only with social recognition, such as facial expressions or perspective taking but signal generation as well. For example, researchers have frequently reported that ASD produces lower facial expressions and a lower magnitude of multiple signal synchronization. In addition to these nonverbal signals, there have been reports on characteristic verbal traits such as frequent use of newly generated words (neologism) or unstoppable talking exclusively on the person's favorite topics within a very narrow range of interests (restricted interest) [7]. To deal with all these characteristics, we need to consider as many multimodal signals as possible while using the flexible estimation power of machine learning.

4.1.1 Monologue Video Dataset

We used a video dataset of monologues collected by Tanaka et al. [8]. This dataset includes 27 videos of talking to a virtual agent on a screen in front of each participant from among nondisabled adults with a mean age of 25.1.

Participants were asked to talk to the virtual agent about positive events they had recently experienced. This task is related to "expressing positive behavior," the first of four fundamental social skills defined by Bellack: expressing positive behavior, listening to others, asking favors, and refusing requests (TELL, LISTEN, ASK, and REFUSE, respectively) [6].

The recording duration was set to one minute. Although a longer talk session might have been better for capturing the characteristic behaviors of users, it would also have been a more challenging task for participants. Some participants reported it was difficult to talk continuously, even for one minute. Therefore, the recording duration was set to one minute to balance these factors.

After the video recording, participants were asked to answer two questionnaires: the Big Five Personality Test and SRS-2. A human annotator transcribed every user's utterances.

4.1.2 Social Responsiveness Scale, 2nd Edition (SRS-2)

SRS-2 is an evaluation metric of the severity of social impairment, and it comprises 65 questions for calculating an overall score and 5 subscales. Although SRS-2 was initially designed to assess potential autism spectrum disorder (ASD) sufferers, it can also differentiate various mental diseases. Furthermore, its effectiveness has been investigated and confirmed not only with disabled people but also with nondisabled people [7]. For this experiment, in addition to the overall score, we also used the social communication subscale, since the overall score includes lifestyle factors such as clothing and bathing, which are not directly related to social communication.

For the overall score distribution, the average and the standard deviation were 65.90 and 19.77, respectively, for males and 61.50 and 21.00 for females. Since the symptomatic population of ASD is gender imbalanced, its cutoff values differ at 65 and 52 for males and females, respectively [9]. Based on these cutoff values, this dataset includes scores in the general population range and those in the ASD range, although participants had never received any clinical diagnosis. Therefore, although it was not planned in advance, these subjects were suitable for this experimental research.

4.1.3 Statistical Features

To compare the effectiveness of multimodal features, we used two different feature sets for this estimation. One is from Takana's work, consisting of 11 features: words per minute, words over six letters, number of fillers, vocal amplitude mean, coefficient of F0 variation, pause percentage, spectral tilt between F1 and F3 (H1A3), smile ratio, and head poses (pitch, yaw, roll) [10]. In this experiment, we set this as the baseline and extended it by adding text features that consider speech contents as well as additional nonverbal features.

To increase the variety of baseline audio features, the proposed model used features from a job interview scoring system [11]. We decided to apply these features to this research because both job interviews and SSTs require similar skills to achieve better performance. When people communicate with others, linguistic speech content and other nonverbal information deliver the speaker's true intentions to listeners. Furthermore, previous research on ASD and schizophrenia patients reported significant differences in audio features such as pause duration and pitch (F0) variability, which enhances our motivation to include audio features in this analysis. These features were calculated with the audio analysis toolkit Praat.[1]

In addition to the smile ratio in baseline, we used signals of action units (AUs) from OpenFace[2] to inject rich information on the subject's facial expression. It is said that facial expressions are essential for communication, and their effectiveness has been reported in previous work. OpenFace's AU recognition evaluates two different attributes: presence and intensity. Presence is a binary attribute indicating whether the AU is detected. In contrast, intensity is a continuous value indicating the strength of the AU's presence, ranging from 0 to 5. Since presence was more stable than intensity in our preliminary experiments, we chose presence as the AU feature for this study. In addition, since the number of video frames differed depending on the given video, we used the average of these presence values for each AU as the input feature to the machine learning model. Moreover, since OpenFace also can extract head-pose information, we calculated the average pose in absolute value and the coefficient of variation for pitch, yaw, and roll.

Regarding text features, we selected word per minute (WPM), vocabulary size, and words with more than six letters, which have been reported as a characteristic in ASD populations. Furthermore, we added filler percentage (Filler %), pronoun percentage (Pronoun %), conjunction percentage (Conj %), and frequency of identical neighboring content words based on previous reports.

4.1.4 BERT-Based Sequential Similarity

In addition to these statistical features, speech content is also vital for analysis. This is especially important for schizophrenia, a symptomatically similar disorder to ASD, showing problematic symptoms labeled "disorganized speech." An extreme example of this is found in Bleuler's book: "I always liked geography. My last teacher in that subject was Professor August A. He was a man with black eyes. I also like black eyes. There are also blue and gray eyes and other sorts, too..." [12]. Although this symptom has been recognized for years, capturing it by automatic calculation has not been easy. Thus, it is necessary to consider the context of the speech. For this purpose, we proposed BERT-based sequential similarity features, named sequential similarity (Seq_sim), to capture this symptom. The following Eq. 1 shows Seq_sim's calculation, where N is the total number of words, Co (A, B) is the cosine similarity between A and B, and embed i is the ith embedding:

$$Seq\_sim = \frac{1}{N}\sum_{i=1}^{N} Cos(embed_{i-1}, embed_i). \tag{1}$$

[1] https://fon.hum.uva.nl/praat/

[2] https://github.com/TadasBaltrusaitis/OpenFace

BERT is a type of neural network initially proposed in the natural language processing field. Compared to previous neural network approaches like Word2Vec, BERT can capture context across an entire input text regardless of its length. Therefore, BERT provides better word-level representation than previous methods like Word2Vec. We used the BERT pre-trained model from the Transformers library (Bert-base-Japanese) for embedding calculations. To investigate the effectiveness of BERT-based features, we also calculated Word2Vec-based features. The score should be high if the user produces only similar words sequentially. This text feature was implemented based on a physician's report that people with ASD tend to use only a limited variety of words compared to nondisabled people. Moreover, we also aimed to capture disorganized speech by using these features. Unlike conventional topic models (e.g., Latent Dirichlet Allocation), this method does not require hyperparameters to define several topic classes.

Interestingly, a series of BERT-based sequential similarities showed a significant correlation with subjective scores on sentence qualities (word choice appropriateness, fluency, sentence structure) [13]. Furthermore, they were significantly correlated with statistical linguistic features (percentage of pronouns, total word counts, dependency distance) as well. These results show the usefulness of BERT-based sequential similarities as an overall quality measure for sentences.

4.1.5 Experiment and Results

As with the previous research by Tanaka, we used linear regression as a machine learning model [10]. More recent models such as LightGBM sometimes show better prediction performance, but this can vary in situations with a limited data amount. For our situation, the number of data is 27, which is very small, so linear regression is suitable with regard to its required data amount and explainability. However, due to the simplicity of linear regression, it can be easily degraded by multicollinearity across different features. To avoid this, we applied a feature selection method based on Pearson's correlation score if the total number of features exceeded 10. We calculated F-statistic values based on Pearson's correlation to sort features in descending order. Then, we filtered all data except for the top 10 relevant features.

All input features were standardized to have an average value of zero and a standard deviation of one. Sometimes, linear regression is used with regularization such as L1, L2, and a combination of L1 and L2 called elastic net. However, such regularizations did not make any improvement in our preliminary experiments. Therefore, no regularization method was adopted. In preparing the features, we found an outlier caused by a failure of the head-pose estimation. Consequently, we eliminated this from the dataset and trained the models using the remaining data of the 26 participants with 67 features each. To deal with the limited size of the dataset, we utilized the leave-one-out cross-validation technique to minimize individuality.

Table 1 shows the results for ASD severity estimation, where SetX indicates feature-setX, select. Indicates feature selection, Correl shows Pearson's correlation score between ground-truth values and estimated values, Correl with * indicates a

Table 1 Results of ASD severity estimation

Name	SRS		Com	
	Correl	RMSE	Correl	RMSE
Set1	0.28	32.13	0.45*	11.33
Set2	0.42*	18.8	0.3	10.54
Set2 with select	0.76*	13.49	0.63*	8.42

significant difference in the test of no correlation, and RMSE indicates root-mean-squared-error.

From the prediction results shown in Table 1, we found that feature-set1 could adequately predict the social communication score because its correlation coefficient was significantly correlated to the ground-truth scores ($p < 0.05$). Surprisingly, despite its limited multimodal features, it demonstrated its predictive ability. This was because the subjective speaking score, the target score used in Tanaka's original research, and the social communication scores were highly correlated, with a coefficient of − 0.39. However, they were not significantly correlated with overall score prediction using feature-set1. This might be because the overall score includes communication aspects of social skills, daily habits, and other non-communicational information, which is not included in the social communication subscale. Compared to feature-set1, feature-set2 with feature selection was more effective in predicting scores with a correlation coefficient of 0.76 for the overall score and 0.63 for the social communication score, implying the effectiveness of the feature selection method.

Focusing on selected features, in both overall score prediction and social communication score prediction, the standard deviation of F0 had the highest coefficient. Moreover, the effectiveness of text features such as vocabulary_size and BERT_content_word was seen only in social communication prediction.

Out of the selected features, F0_SD had the highest feature coefficient of linear regression. In previous research, the authors reported that an irregularity of F0 movement was found in ASD patients and schizophrenia patients as explained in Sect. 4.1.4. The results from this experiment support those earlier findings. Interestingly, the effectiveness of text features was only seen in the results of social communication score prediction, not in overall score prediction. These results indicate that text content (i.e., what was said) was unimportant for overall score prediction.

4.2 *Social Skill Estimation*

As we explained above, understanding the meaning of multimodal signals is necessary for social communications. Despite its importance, the automatic recognition of this meaning is quite challenging, since humans have extraordinary abilities to infer the ambiguous intentions of each social behavior, which is technically very difficult

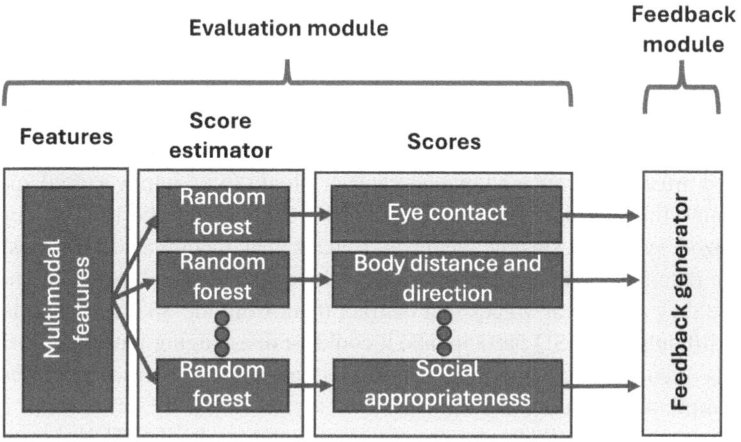

Fig. 1 Schematic of our evaluation-feedback pipeline of social skill scores

to achieve in a system. To fill this gap, we attempted to build automatic social skills estimation models using multimodal signals with machine learning techniques.

Compared to previous visual feedback directly corresponding to feature values, our system estimated social skills with multimodal machine learning models to consider complex skills based on the interaction among features. We also developed an automated evaluation-feedback pipeline with a summary feedback strategy inspired by experienced SST trainers. To deal with complex evaluations by human trainers, as the core of our automated quantitative evaluation, we set the following seven component scores: eye contact, body direction/distance, facial expression, vocal variation, clarity, fluency, and social appropriateness. Our system consists of two modules: (1) an evaluation module for seven-component social-skill-score estimation with machine learning models and (2) a feedback module that generates positive/corrective feedback language based on the seven estimated component scores (Fig. 1). In the latter part of this chapter, we focus on the first module's score estimation. Refer to the earlier work for details of both modules [14].

4.2.1 SST Dataset

We used a human–human and a human-agent SST dataset of 276 sessions, including 19 healthy controls, 15 people with schizophrenia, and 16 people with ASD [14]. We combined data from the control and clinical groups to train the social skill estimation models as a way to maximize the training dataset size because machine learning methods require much data for better estimation stability in general. This also makes it possible to extend our system target to the general population. For example, our social skills training system should be helpful for job-hunting students or people with difficulty communicating with their co-workers. Furthermore, the participation of the clinical groups can also absorb the skewed distribution of social skill scores since the control group's scores were skewed toward the better side. In contrast, the scores of the clinical groups were generally on the worse side. Therefore, a mixed data group provides less biased training of the machine learning models. As data from clinical populations, we combined ASD and SZ symptomatic groups, since there are reports that they share several symptomatically similar characteristics such as flat or blunted affect (e.g., reduced eye contact) or alogia (e.g., impoverished speech). At the same time, these two-group data collections can also be used to generate personalized, symptom-specific feedback. Bellack et al. recommended using shorter and more precise feedback for people with schizophrenia who have hallucinations [6]. Since they often hear voices that distract them from the SST, finding where to focus is difficult. For ASD participants, it could be disengaging feedback if trainers frequently mentioned exaggerated gestures or facial expressions, since these are major symptomatic characteristics.

The dataset includes SST sessions of four role-play tasks (LISTEN: listening to others, TELL: conveying positive feelings, ASK: requesting from others, DECLINE: declining a request) for each participant based on Bellack's definition of the four basic social skills [6]. Some participants repeated SST sessions using the same task two or even three times for further improvement. The length of each session ranged from 30 s to 2 min. The dataset includes 168 sessions (LISTEN: 43, TELL: 34, ASK: 46, DECLINE: 45). Since it is better to have a larger dataset to boost the robustness of the machine learning training, we combined additional human-agent interaction data with a similar recording protocol from our series of SST automation research. Consequently, our extended dataset for the machine learning models comprised 276 sessions (LISTEN: 70, TELL: 61, ASK: 73, and DECLINE: 72). We used the core dataset of 168 sessions for the feedback's content analysis and the extended dataset of 276 sessions for the machine learning training. For more details, including recruitment conditions, please refer to Sect. 3.

4.2.2 Feedback Content Analysis

Since the analytic components of SST by human trainers were not clear for adaptation to automation, we started by analyzing the contents of feedback by professionals. Furthermore, feedback analysis is also necessary to achieve better training outcomes. According to self-efficacy theory, people who receive efficacious feedback will be motivated to act, whereas those whose self-efficacy is lowered by feedback will lose motivation. Therefore, how to give feedback is critical to SST outcomes; unfortunately, there is no concrete SST feedback method. For this reason, we analyzed the feedback characteristics of experienced trainers toward developing an automatic system.

As a result, we identified 37 feedback types based on the trainers' feedback. The top 10 most frequent feedback types accounted for 71% of all 37 types. The number of positive feedback types was always higher than that of corrective ones. Four of these top 10 feedback types (Gave reasons, Concrete speech content, Proposed alternatives, and Checked whether they had time to talk) involved speech content (linguistic features). In contrast, the remaining six types involved verbal and nonverbal skills (paralinguistic features).

Based on these results, we constructed input features for social skill estimation. For example, we measured appropriate facial expressions by using the intensity values of the facial action units of OpenFace as input to the evaluation models. Note that this "appropriateness" depends on each SST task, which can be represented, for example, by smiley faces for "expressing positive feelings" or contrite faces for "declining requests." We also measured Concrete speech content by counting the content words (e.g., nouns, verbs, adjectives, nominal adjectives, adverbs) of each user's utterances. To capture expressing apology and declining clearly, we prepared a set of keywords to judge whether the user showed appropriate expression for each task.

4.2.3 Multimodal Features

We calculated 55 automated multimodal features to estimate their scores as shown in Table 2. In detail, we used 11 features from the text modality, 2 from the audio modality, 39 from the facial image modality, and 3 from the Kinect body point modality. Those features were initially designed to estimate discrete feedback labels by experienced SST trainers in feedback content analysis. However, that resulted in poor performance, and we assumed that the annotation was too sparse (most annotations were 0), since the distribution was highly imbalanced. Accordingly, we changed the estimation target to a subjective component score of social skills.

Compared to the feature sets described in Sects. 4.1.3 and 4.1.4, although we used several overlapping features, there were significant differences, as follows, because the system's goal is to achieve SST feedback, which needs to be interpretable. First, we modified the variations of BERT-based sequential similarities for the text modality and replaced other statistical measures except for WPM. In addition, we kept only average voice intensity and coefficient of F0 variation for the audio modality. Although detailed audio analyses provide precise information that humans could not recognize in general, those precise features were unnecessary for imitating feedback by human SST trainers. Therefore, we implemented the two features based on the SST feedback content from the SST trainers. We added the standard deviation of body joint positions to capture body gestures in the SST interactions and thus extended the previous feature set for the visual modality.

4.2.4 Social Skill Estimation Models

To investigate the best model for our problem, we started with a comparison of prediction models including partial least square (PLS) regression, SVR, random forest, dense neural network, and variational autoencoder (VAE) for the regression model. Since SVR showed better performance than LASSO regression in Naim's study, we

Table 2 Input features used for proposed automated evaluation models

Feature name	Explanation
BERT_self_self_sent	Sentence-level intra-person BERT-based seq-similarity
BERT_self_self_cont	Content-word-level intra-person BERT-based seq-similarity
BERT_self_inter_sent	Sentence-level inter-person BERT-based seq-similarity
BERT_self_inter_cont	Content-word-level inter-person BERT-based seq-similarity
Num_content	Number of content words
Thanks_flag	Binary flag for the presence of appreciative language
Sorry_flag	Binary flag for the presence of apologetic language
Explicit_refuse_flag	Binary flag for presence of explicit refusal language
Num_backchannel	Number of backchannels
Init_cue_flag	Binary flag for presence of initialization cue words
WPM	Words per minute
Ave_voice_int	Average voice intensity
CV_voice_f0	Coefficient of variation of F0
Smile_freq	Percentage of smile frequency ranging from 0.0 to 1.0
Head_mean	Mean value of head poses (treated *x*, *y*, *z* values in a same axis)
Head_CV	Coefficient of variation of head poses
Num_nod	Number of nods
Mutual_smile	Percentage of mutual smile frequency ranging from 0.0 to 1.0
AU(XX)_r_(mean, CV)	Mean intensity and coefficient of variation of facial action unit 01, 02, 04, 06, 07, 09, 10, 12, 15, 17, 20, 23, 25, 26, 45 ranging from 0.0 to 1.0
Gesture_all_CV	Coefficient of variation of all body joints
Gesture_upper_CV	Coefficient of variation of upper body joints
Gesture_arm_CV	Coefficient of variation of arm body joints

decided to include it. Random forest is known for its over-fit robustness for small-sized datasets. Furthermore, a recent study proved its stability in learning theoretically; therefore, we adopted it for this study. Additionally, we added PLS regression and the "VAE for regression" model, which can compress sparse information (e.g., our multimodal features) to a lower-dimensional space. We also attempted to experimentally construct an original neural network, since recent neural network methods have shown promising results. PLS, SVR and random forest cannot estimate multiple scores simultaneously, so we trained separate models for each component skill score. On the other hand, we trained them in a simultaneous multi-output format because neural networks can simultaneously estimate various scores. This should be more suitable for social skill estimation by considering inter-score interactions, which is impossible to achieve using a single-output format. As an additional experiment with the winning model, we ran an abrasion study on feature modalities to investigate the effects on each fundamental social skill.

Since each person has a unique style of using social skills, producing a wide variety of styles, we must consider individuality effects to prevent data leakage in machine learning. For instance, one participant expressed their gratitude with hand gestures showing surprise and a smiling face, while another used a high tone of voice. Although machine learning methods can estimate ambiguous values, they tend to over-fit training samples when the dataset size is small and includes a participant with a characteristic communication style. Therefore, to prevent this problem, we employed leave-one-participant-out cross-validation in our training. We first selected one participant as test data, followed by selecting another participant as validation data. We used the remaining data as the training set.

Table 3 shows the model comparison results for the estimation of social skill scores, where Correl. indicates Spearman's correlation coefficient and values with * indicate a significant correlation in the no-correlation test. The table shows the component-merged task scores (R^2 and Spearman's correlation coefficient) to compare the model performances at the abstract level.

We confirmed that every model achieved significantly correlated predictions for all of the tasks, although there are differences in the levels of the statistics. Regarding R^2, deep learning-based models showed lower scores than conventional methods. This result might be caused by the limited data size, where millions of data are usually used for neural network training to achieve better performance. For this reason, researchers using small-sized datasets have frequently reported that conventional methods show the most promising results. In our case, the random forest model performed best for all the tasks with R^2 scores over 0.13 and correlation coefficients over 0.38. We believe this result can be explained by the fact that tree-based models generally work well for interpolation settings, and our target social skill scores were within a limited range of 1–5 with several 100-ordered data samples.

Table 3 Model comparison

Model	LISTEN		TELL		ASK		DECLINE	
	R^2	Correl	R^2	Correl	R^2	Correl	R^2	Correl
PLS	− 0.71	0.20*	− 0.78	0.10*	− 0.42	0.32*	− 0.24	0.47*
SVR_rbf	0.15	0.42*	0.13	0.37*	0.13	0.42*	0.09	0.38*
Random forest	0.13	0.38*	0.16	0.39*	0.2	0.45*	0.16	0.42*
Neural network	− 1.76	0.31*	− 2.27	0.34*	− 1.14	0.31*	− 1.76	0.31*
VAE for regression	− 1.1	0.33*	− 1.79	0.36*	− 0.86	0.44*	− 0.88	0.49*

Tables 4 and 5 show the results of the social-skill score estimation, where Correl. denotes Spearman's correlation between the ground-truth and the estimated score. Scores with * in the Correl. column showed a significant correlation in the no-correlation test ($p < 0.05$).

In each component skill score level with random forest, although most results showed a significant correlation, some components needed further improvement. Facial expression, for instance, failed to estimate the scores for the ASK and DECLINE tasks. The difference between successful tasks (LISTEN, TELL) and failed tasks (ASK, DECLINE) is the complexity of the facial expressions for each one. Since the discussion themes of the successful tasks were simple, they did not flip from positive to negative topics. We set only positive themes for the agent utterances in the LISTEN task and asked users to share their positive feelings in the TELL task. Therefore, the facial expression could only be a neutral or a smiling face, which was easy to measure. On the other hand, the failed tasks needed positive or negative facial expressions depending on the discussion phases. For example, the ASK task needs a contrite facial expression at the beginning. However, after the agent accepts the user's request, the user can choose to express a thankful feeling with a smile to continue to talk with an apologetic face. Since either expression could be correct, measuring the appropriateness is technically challenging depending on the dialogue context. One reason for this technical hurdle is that our current estimation system cannot accurately handle the synchronized timing of each multimodal feature, since we averaged the features across all of the time frames of the session video. We need to change our approach to sequential models for such a timing-sensitive feature to capture its synchrony adequately. Another challenge is capturing an appropriate representation

Table 4 Results of social-skill score estimation (1 of 2)

Task	Label	R^2	RMSE	Correl
LISTEN	Eye contact	0.01	0.7	0.14
	Body direction and distance	0	0.71	0.22*
	Facial expression	0.04	1.18	0.26*
	Vocal variation	0.04	1.23	0.26*
	Clarity	– 0.02	1.12	0.05
	Fluency	0.13	1.01	0.38*
	Social appropriateness	0.18	1	0.47*
TELL	Eye contact	0.11	0.57	0.29*
	Body direction and distance	0.19	0.65	0.45*
	Facial expression	0.15	1.26	0.37*
	Vocal variation	0.12	1.05	0.31*
	Clarity	0.01	1.08	0.13
	Fluency	0.17	0.9	0.33*
	Social appropriateness	0.04	1.09	0.04

* denotes significant correlation in no-correlation test

Table 5 Results of social-skill score estimation (2 of 2)

Task	Label	R^2	RMSE	Correl
ASK	Eye contact	0.06	0.82	0.22
	Body direction and distance	0.11	0.51	0.33*
	Facial expression	0.03	1.27	0.21
	Vocal variation	0.09	1.16	0.24*
	Clarity	0.4	0.79	0.68*
	Fluency	0.03	1.07	0.24*
	Social appropriateness	0.34	0.93	0.63*
DECLINE	Eye contact	-0.06	1.05	0.04
	Body direction and distance	0.14	0.74	0.39*
	Facial expression	0.03	1.44	0.19
	Vocal variation	0.07	1.53	0.28*
	Clarity	0.07	1.66	0.33*
	Fluency	0.12	1.33	0.38*
	Social appropriateness	0.15	1.26	0.36*

* denotes significant correlation in no-correlation test

of the speech contents. To deal with this problem, cutting-edge NLP methods, such as speech-graph representations, are required [15].

Table 6 shows the R^2 scores in the modality ablation study with the random forest model. Only a drop in the visual modality led to a performance decrease of 0.12 for the TELL task and 0.10 for the ASK task in R^2. This implies the importance of visual information for TELL and ASK. These results are intuitively understandable because these tasks require more expressive skills than LISTEN or DECLINE. Therefore, the model's performance greatly decreased by reducing such visual information as facial expressions and body gestures.

Table 6 R^2 of ablation study on modalities

Feature modality	LISTEN	TELL	ASK	DECLINE
V + A + L	0.13	0.16	0.2	0.16
A + L	0.13	0.04	0.1	0.2
V + L	0.11	0.17	0.21	0.16
V + A	0.14	0.12	0.17	0.11

5 Future Perspective

As introduced in this chapter, researchers have worked on automatic behavior modeling using machine learning models with multimodal signals, including our work on ASD severity estimation and social skill estimation. Although behavior modeling is possible in some limited situations, there are still several technical difficulties to be solved. In closing this chapter, we need to clarify these points.

Social communications are time-sensitive, so they should be well-aligned to provide good communication. Therefore, it is more suitable to assess them sequentially with sequential models such as LSTM or Transformer architectures. Due to limited training data, we used conventional machine learning models such as linear regression, random forest, and PLS regression for this study's experiments. Since recording human–human SST imposes a heavy workload, it is not feasible to increase the size of our dataset. However, this problem might be overcome by annotating score labels for existing human–human interaction datasets such as NoXi, which is a more realistic approach than creating a huge social skills training dataset from scratch, which would require the total devotion of many clinicians. Furthermore, the recent trends in large language models (LLMs), which are evolving to provide multimodal and sequential capabilities without external data for fine-tuning (e.g., GPT-4o,[3] Gemini 1.5 Pro[4]), will make it possible to solve problems of limited data size, like ours, through precise time-aligned precise analysis and a better understanding of interactive behaviors. As a first step toward LLM integration, feedback generation from estimated social skills scores might be a feasible choice.

Since there is no conventional SST evaluation metric, we used seven component scores annotated by experienced trainers to develop the proposed social skills evaluation models. However, these scores are task-specific because essential social skills can vary depending on the social context, even for the same evaluation target. To overcome this limitation, we must use generic metrics. Although the question of which evaluation metric to use remains a controversial issue, the social performance rating scale (SPRS) might be another choice. It should be noted, however, that despite its validated generalizability across tasks and cultures, it still depends on subjective annotation. Therefore, finding and implementing an objective metric would be better for reliable evaluations.

Even in this era of large language models (LLMs), there is no doubt that multimodal behavior modeling is still a quite difficult task to solve. With the power of *truly* multimodal LLMs (using three or more modalities, not only two), we hope that the difficulties of social communication will disappear, or that those suffering from them will be more accepted by society than under the current situation. How to implement this technology or use it effectively might be the next target of multimodal behavior modeling research.

[3] https://openai.com/index/hello-gpt-4o/

[4] https://blog.google/technology/ai/google-gemini-next-generation-model-february-2024/

Acknowledgements This chapter was mainly modified and extended from the PhD thesis of the first author at Nara Institute of Science and Technology for this publication. Funding was provided by the Core Research for Evolutionary Science and Technology (Grant No. JPMJCR19A5).

References

1. P. Short, Social Communication: Conversation and Mass Media. In: Society and Gender. Palgrave, London. (1992) https://doi.org/10.1007/978-1-349-15168-4_7
2. F.F. Steen et al. (2018) Toward an infrastructure for data-driven multimodal communication research. Linguist. Vanguard, vol. 4, no. 1. https://doi.org/10.1515/lingvan-2017-0041
3. X. Alameda-Pineda et al., Multimodal behavior analysis in the wild: an introduction. Multimodal Behav. Anal. Wild (2019). https://doi.org/10.1016/B978-0-12-814601-9.00011-0
4. T.M. Fischer et al. Communication Analysis through Visual Analytics: Current Practices, Challenges, and New Frontiers. 2022 IEEE Visualization in Data Science (VDS), (2022) https://doi.org/10.1109/VDS57266.2022.00006
5. T. Sasaki, Validation of revised role-play test towards social skills evaluation for schizophrenia Kaiteiban rooru purei tesuto no sinraisei oyobi datousei no kentou—tougousittyoushou no syakaiseikatsuginou no hyouka ni mukete (in japanese). Clin. Psychiatry Seishin Igaku (in Japanese) **48**(11), 1191–1198 (2006)
6. A.S. Bellack et al. Social Skills Training for Schizophrenia: A Step-by-Step Guide. Guilford Press, 2 edition. (2004)
7. J.N. Constantino et al. Social Responsiveness Scale, Second Edition (SRS-2). Western Psychological Services. (2012)
8. H. Tanaka et al., Analysis of conversational listening skills toward agent-based social skills training. J. Multimodal User Interfaces **14**(1), 73–82 (2020)
9. R. Takei et al. Verification of the utility of the social responsiveness scale for adults in non-clinical and clinical adult populations in japan. BMC Psychiatry, 14(302), (2014)
10. H. Tanaka et al., Embodied conversational agents for multimodal automated social skills training in people with autism spectrum disorders. PLoS ONE **12**(8), 1–15 (2017)
11. I. Naim et al. Automated analysis and prediction of job interview performance. IEEE Trans. Affect. Comput. (2015)
12. E. Bleuler, Dementia Praecox, or the Group of Schizophrenias. New York: International Universities Press, (1950)
13. T. Saga et al. (2022) Multimodal prediction of social responsiveness score with BERT-based text features, IEICE Trans. Inform. Syst. Human Commun., E105-D, 3, 578–586 (2022)
14. T. Saga et al., Automatic evaluation-feedback system for automated social skills training. Sci. Rep. **13**, 6856 (2023)
15. N.B. Mota et al., Speech graphs provide a quantitative measure of thought disorder in psychosis. PLoS ONE **7**(4), 1–9 (2012)
16. S. Kawano et al., Multimodal persuasive dialogue corpus using a teleoperated android. Proc. Interspeech **2022**, 2308–2312 (2022). https://doi.org/10.21437/Interspeech.2022-565
17. L. Hemamou et al., Hirenet: A hierarchical attention model for the automatic analysis of asynchronous video job interviews. Proceed. AAAI Conf. Artif. Intell. **33**(01), 573–581 (2019)

Introduces the Virtual Agent

Multimodal Adaptive Behavior Generation During Human–Agent Interaction

Jieyeon Woo, Catherine Achard, and Catherine Pelachaud

Abstract Interaction consists of verbal exchange as well as multimodal social signals. Multimodality is essential in communicating fruitfully by sending implicit and explicit information. When conversing, multimodal signals are transferred back and forth between interlocutors. Via this transfer, interlocutors constantly adapt their behaviors to those of their interlocutors. Virtual agents, which look and act like humans, should also consider the multimodal and adaptive aspect of the interaction they build with the users. In this chapter, we elaborate on adaptive behavior evaluation methods, multimodal adaptive behavior generation modeling, and the effect of a virtual agent providing real-time adaptive behaviors for cognitive behavioral therapy (CBT).

1 Introduction

Information is transferred from one person to another and vice versa via multimodal signals such as speech content, gestures, and prosody. Through this two-way exchange, sending and receiving, interlocutors constantly adapt their behaviors in response to each other [1–4]. Such adaptation is continuous, dynamic, and reciprocal which is also referred to as reciprocal adaptation [5–8]. The endowment of adaptation to virtual agents can make them more social and engaging, and perceived as natural and human-like. It is interesting to learn how adaptive capacity could be endowed and also to check whether such improvement could be brought to virtual agents that serve for medical treatment such as cognitive behavioral therapy (CBT).

J. Woo (✉)
Korea Institute of Machinery and Materials, Daejeon, South Korea
e-mail: jywoo@kimm.re.kr

C. Achard
ISIR, Sorbonne University, Paris, France
e-mail: achard@isir.upmc.fr

C. Pelachaud
CNRS, ISIR, Sorbonne University, Paris, France
e-mail: pelachaud@isir.upmc.fr

S. Nakamura (ed.), *Multimodal Interaction Technologies for Training Affective Social Skills*, https://doi.org/10.1007/978-981-96-1313-7_8

Before investigating the adaptation modeling or the result evaluation, it is critical to design the adaptation assessment methods. We will thus first look into the interaction dataset followed up by the methods of evaluating the adaptation within an interaction including reciprocal adaptation measures. Then, we will introduce our modeling of multimodal reciprocally adaptive behavior generation, the ASAP model [6]. As it is important for agents to act as interactive partners and continuously adapt their behaviors in real-time, we will present our real-time interactive and adaptive agent, the IAVA system [9], and show the effectiveness of adaptive virtual agents for the application to CBT.

2 Interaction Dataset

We chose the NoXi database [10] consisting of human–human interactions for our empirical study concerning adaptive behavior evaluation, adaptive behavior modeling, and real-time adaptive virtual agent system perception and generation.

NoXi contains screen-mediated face-to-face interactions which are natural dyadic conversations talking about a common topic. A pair of participants each with different roles, either expert or novice, are in each interaction video. The corpus consists of three parts depending on the recording location (France, Germany, and UK). For our work, we only use the French recordings (excluding the recordings from Germany, and UK) which are made up of 21 dyadic interactions performed by 28 participants with a total duration of 7h22min.

The interaction dataset is multimodal in the sense that the video recording provides visual and audio information. We obtain nonverbal behavior features for both interacting participants through feature extraction. For each time step, the visual and audio features, listed in Table 1, are extracted using open-source toolkits of OpenFace and openSMILE, respectively.

To clean up the data, we process the visual and audio features separately.

We start by processing the visual data on the extracted visual feature. We first filter out unsuccessful extractions as there are some moments where OpenFace extracts the features with low accuracy extracting wrong feature values. We interpolate to fill in the dropped values and smooth out the feature data by applying a median filter (win = 7). Then, different scaling techniques, normalization, and standardization methods depicted in Table 2, are applied depending on the characteristics of each feature. The scaling technique of Type 1 is applied to the head rotations, head translations, and gaze as their values are centered around the mean with a unit standard deviation. For facial AUs, the Type 2 scaling technique is employed as their intensity values range from 0 to 5.

The audio processing starts with the denoising of the audio files, removing surrounding sound, via Audacity's noise reduction. The denoised audio is used to extract the audio features. The extracted audio features are processed with their corresponding scaling technique similar to the preprocessing of visual features as found in Table 2. The scaling techniques applied to different audio features are as follows:

Table 1 Extracted features from the NoXi corpus

Feature			Description
Visual	Head rotation	R_x	Head rotation around the x axis
		R_y	Head rotation around the y axis
		R_x	Head rotation around the z axis
	Head translation	T_x	Head translation around the x axis
		T_y	Head translation around the y axis
		T_z	Head translation around the z axis
	Gaze (or eye movement)	G_x	Gaze around the x axis
		G_y	Gaze around the y axis
	Facial action units	AU1	Inner brow raiser
		AU2	Outer brow raiser
		AU4	Brow lowerer
		AU5	Upper lid raiser
		AU6	Cheek raiser
		AU7	Lid tightener
		AU12	Lip corner puller for smile
		AU15	Lip corner depressor
Audio	Fundamental frequency (or pitch)	F0	Predominant frequency representing the speech quality
	Loudness		Speech intensity from the auditory spectra
	Voicing probability		Speech presence probability expressed as a probability score in the range of 0 to 1
	Mel-Frequency-Cepstral Coefficients (MFCC)		Representation of the short-term power spectrum of a sound; represented by 13 MFCC features (0–12)

Table 2 Scaling technique types corresponding to each feature

	Scaling technique	Feature (s)
Type 1	$\frac{f-\mu}{\sigma}$	$R_{x,y,z}$, $T_{x,y,z}$, $G_{x,y,z}$, and MFCCs (1–12)
Type 2	$\frac{f}{f_{max}}$	AUs(1,2,4,5,6,7,12,15) and F0
Type 3	$\frac{f}{f_{max}} * \alpha$	Loudness
Type 4	$\frac{f-f_{min}}{f_{max}-f_{min}}$	MFCC0

Type 1 is applied to the 12 MFCCs (1–12) showing data centers around a mean and different standard deviations of which we want to scale to 1. Type 2 is applied to the pitch (F0) ranging from 0 to each speaker's maximum pitch level. Type 3 is applied to loudness also ranging from 0 to each speaker's maximum loudness value with different standard deviations. To respond to the difference in standard deviation, the standardization method (Type 3) includes a multiplication with α which allows the different values of the same feature to share the same standard deviation value. Type 4 is applied to MFCC0 consisting of values varying between a minimum and maximum value. All the features are adjusted to 25 fps for our study.

3 Evaluation of Adaptive Behavior

Research around virtual agents mostly focuses on developing the agent's behavior by improving the social, engagement, naturalness, and human-likeliness aspects. While it is important to create such behavior, it is also essential to evaluate the behavior quality.

The task of evaluating the agent's quality is in fact challenging. Notably, human–agent interactions are generally evaluated subjectively via surveys but it is not evident to objectively evaluate them. Virtual agents interact with their human users in a similar fashion to humans within an interaction. As such, the assessment of the interaction quality must be done on both sides: at the agent's side and at the interaction level considering the human interlocutor.

During an interaction, various social signals are emitted and perceived. Among the different signals, the smile plays an important role in human interaction. Even the single presence of a smile can express various information, such as the state of affect and engagement as well as the intrinsic nature, to the interacting partner disregarding the social context [11]. In this regard, by looking into the effect of smiling during interactions we can investigate the quality of the adaptation taking place.

In a conversation, interlocutors constantly adapt their behavior but this adapted behavior does not signify that they will always show an explicit response by emitting a signal. Interacting participants may or may not respond to each other's behavior. We focus on measuring reciprocal adaptation via synchrony patterns and entrainment loops. Via the proposal of our reciprocal adaptation measures [5] we capture synchrony patterns when participants respond or do not respond to each other's behaviors. Unlike previous measures which consider the absence of response as an error (e.g., correlation measures and DTW) or ignore them (recurrent analysis), we also take into account the absence of response as it may also convey important information about the interaction.

Via our new measures of adaptation, which assess the synchrony and entrainment loop of dyads, we measure the interaction adaptation and study the impact of the absence of response. We hold a specific interest in measuring the adaption of human behavior during an interaction notably via their smile signals.

3.1 Synchrony Measures

To learn from times when there is an absence of response, we propose new synchrony measures for dyadic pairs which also capture the absence of response. Our synchrony measures capture both synced pairs and unsynced pairs as illustrated in Fig. 1. Synced pairs are detected while tolerating time swift, dilation, deletion, and insertion. For unsynced pairs, we divided them into two types: addition (when a signal is produced by oneself without the reaction of the other interlocutor) and suppression (when a signal is produced by the other interlocutor without the reaction of oneself) of signals.

Inspired by edit distance or Levenshtein distance, we also use the concepts of insertion (i.e., addition of unsynced pairs) and deletion (i.e., suppression of unsynced pairs) of the edit distance (see Fig. 1).

The synchrony is evaluated via signal activation obtained from continuous values after binarization and via subsequence extraction of active signals. For smile activation values, we binarize their continuous intensity values with the threshold of 1.5/5 (smile action unit AU12 is measured within the range of 0–5) which is the manually identified minimal intensity for a smile activation.

Each active signal subsequence is segmented via its starting (s) and ending (e) timing as shown in Fig. 2. Two subsequences, each from interlocutors PA and PB, are identified to be synchronized or paired (i.e., synced pair) if:

$$|e_A - e_B| + |s_A - s_B| \leq \text{threshold}$$

where s_A and s_B are the starting time points and e_A and e_B are the ending time points of subsequences A (from PA) and subsequences B (from PB), respectively, and the threshold is set to twice the time delay (2–4 s [12]). Signals from PA and PB are still perceived as being mimicry.

Both paired and unpaired subsequences (i.e., pairs) of persons PA and PB, illustrated in Fig. 1, are considered for the synchrony estimation. They can be captured with the following equations.

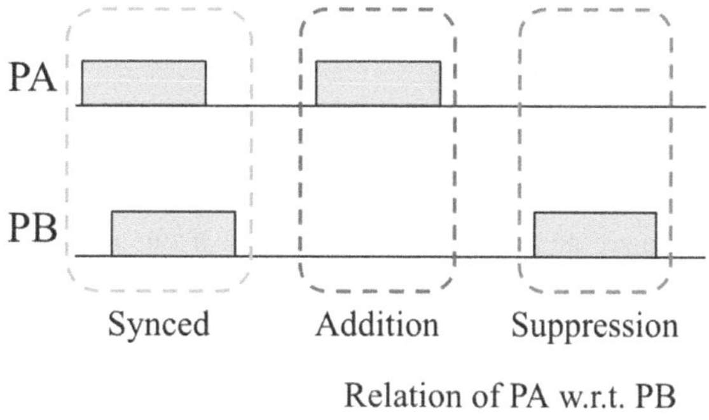

Fig. 1 Illustration of synced and unsynced pairs (i.e., addition and suppression) between two interlocutors PA and PB for person A and person B, respectively

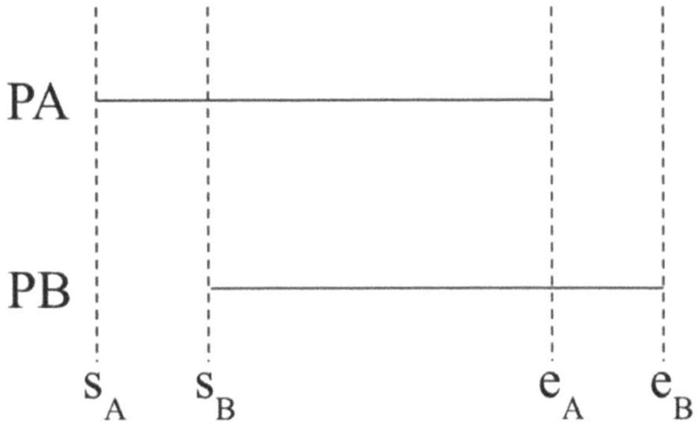

Fig. 2 Illustration of subsequences that are synchronized or paired

$$\text{PA\&PB} = \frac{nb.\text{ of synced pairs}}{\text{total } nb.\text{ of events}}$$
$$\text{PA\&}\neg\text{PB} = \frac{nb.\text{ of unpaired subseq.}s(\text{seq}A|\text{seq}B)}{\text{total } nb.\text{ of events}}$$
$$\text{PB\&}\neg\text{PA} = \frac{nb.\text{ of unpaired subseq.}s(\text{seq}B|\text{seq}A)}{\text{total } nb.\text{ of } events}$$

where the total number of events is the sum of the number of synced and unpaired pairs (i.e., unsynced pairs corresponding to addition and suppression cases) of both persons PA and PB.

Each measure renders a probability that corresponds to the following:

- PA&PB: PA and PB are responding to each other;
- PA&¬PB: PA is actively sending a signal but not PB;
- PB&¬PA: PB is actively sending a signal but not PA.

In the case of a smile, PA&PB indicates that both persons PA and PB are smiling simultaneously or with a small delay (corresponding to the reacting time) representing the sync between PA and PB. Concerning PA&¬PB and PB&¬PA, only a single person, PA or PB, respectively, is sending a signal (PA smiles and PB does not smile, and vice versa). In both cases, PA and PB are not in sync.

3.2 Entrainment Loop Measure

When we adapt our behavior to that of our interlocutor, we change our behavior after perceiving our interlocutor's social signal. This could be thought of as a simple one-way process like an action-reaction process in which the interlocutor's action triggers the reaction (i.e., adaptation) of oneself. Nevertheless, the adaptation is a continuous two-way (i.e., loop) process in which even our reaction can retrigger the reaction of our interlocutor. This looped process is called an entrainment loop. In the case of the smile signal, the smile of person PA can entrain the smile of person

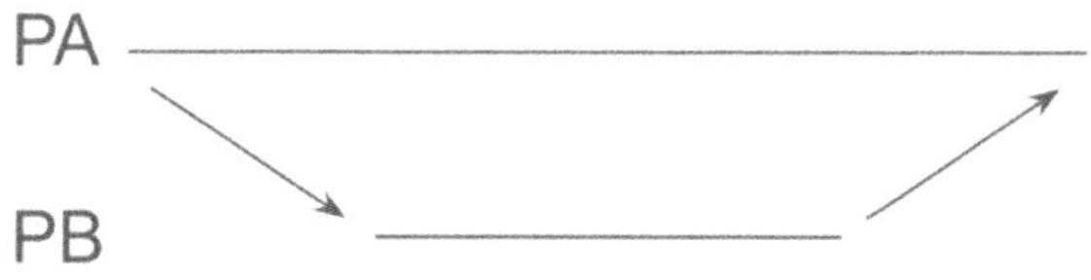

Fig. 3 Entrainment loop Type 1: a continuous smile of PA in [5]

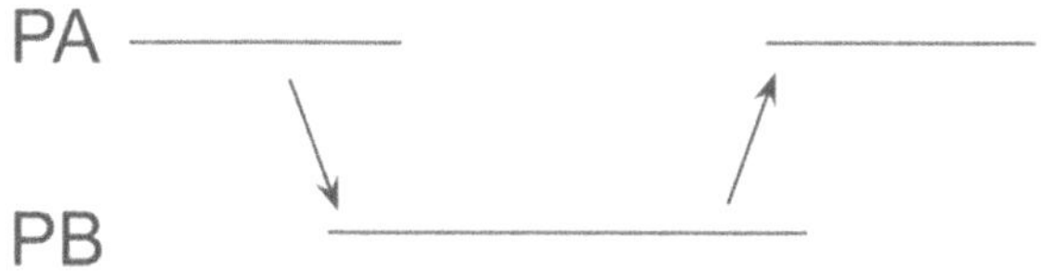

Fig. 4 Entrainment loop Type 2: a repeated smile of PA with overlap in [5]

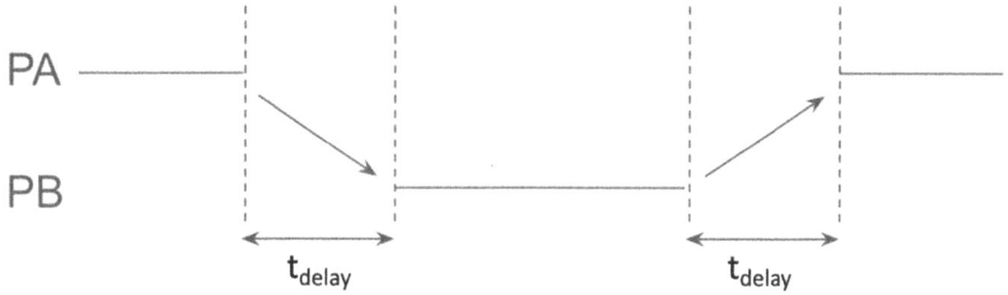

Fig. 5 Entrainment loop Type 2: a repeated smile of PA within the time delay t_{delay}. (*Modified version of the original figure in [5]: Time delay of 4s in [5] noted as t_{delay}.)

PB which can also entrain PA to continue to smile or to smile again within a certain time delay and vice versa.

The entrainment loop consists of two types:

- Type 1: continuous smile, shown in Fig. 3;
- Type 2: repeated smile with an overlap or within a certain time delay (i.e., mimicry delay [12]), shown in Figs. 4 and 5, respectively.

4 Multimodal Reciprocally Adaptive Behavior Generation

Virtual agent research aims to enhance users' experience by improving the agent's naturalness and human-likeliness. To attain this aim, we want the agent to behave naturally like humans do. Looking into human behaviors, behaviors are made up of continuous values that evolve over time. For example, focusing on human motion, we can note that the body landmark positions change smoothly in time. Thus, ensuring the production of continuous behaviors by looking at their temporal continuity is also critical for natural human-like behavior. While it is crucial for behavior motions to be continuous for our research, behaviors should also be coherent (i.e., appropriate) and in sync with those shown by the interactant. Moreover, as virtual agents are designed for human users, it is critical for them to be engaging so that they can grab and maintain the user's attention and interest.

For our study, we focus on producing appropriate agent behavior strengthening the aspects of naturalness and human-likeliness while also raising the user's engagement and synchrony by endowing the agent with the capacity of reciprocal adaptation.

4.1 ASAP Architecture

We introduce the modeling of reciprocal adaptation concentrating on the modelization of interpersonal temporality, multimodality, and behavior continuity. Our proposed Augmented Self-Attention Pruning (ASAP) model [6] renders natural and human-like behaviors, as both listener and speaker, that are coherent, engaging, and in sync with the interlocutor.

ASAP model architecture, illustrated in Fig. 6, consists of three key techniques: data augmentation technique, self-attention pruning, and autoregressive adaptive online prediction. The main advantages of each technique are as follows.

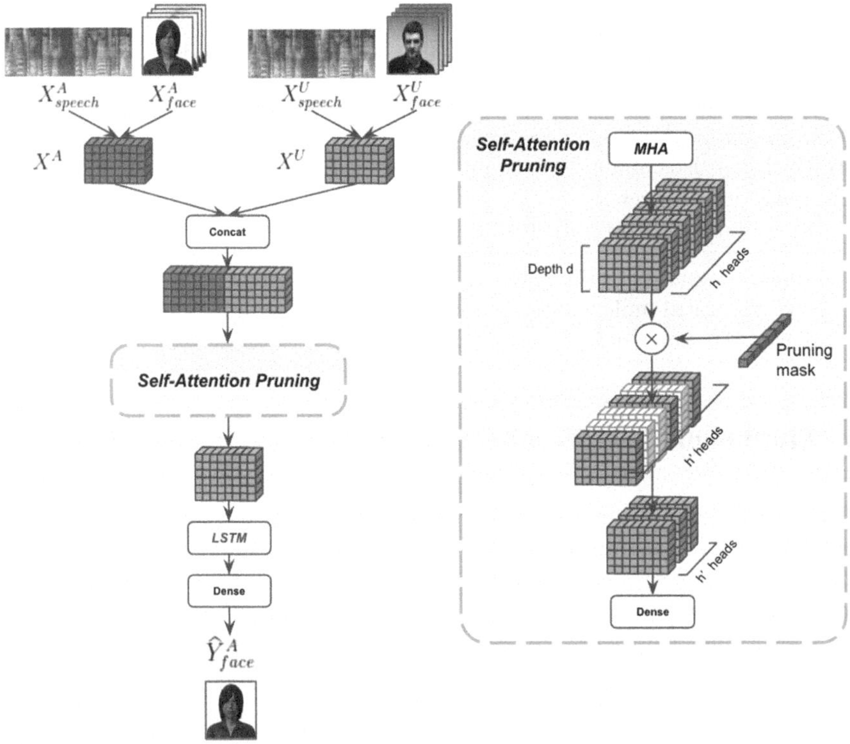

Fig. 6 ASAP (Augmented Self-Attention Pruning) [6] model architecture

- Data augmentation technique: learning from both interactants. This allows the training with a limited amount of data;
- Self-attention pruning: selection of key features within the interaction from multimodal dyadic information;
- Autoregressive adaptive online prediction: generation of continuous agent nonverbal behaviors.

The ASAP model takes the speech X_{speech} and the facial gestures X_{face} of the previous 100 frames (t-99:t) of both the agent (A) and the user (U) to learn the interpersonal relationship (i.e., reciprocal adaptation) between them. The virtual agent's behavior (i.e., facial gesture) for the next frame at $t+1$ $\hat{Y}^A_{\text{face}}$ is generated. To infer the next agent's behavior, we feed back the predicted agent's behavior and the ground truth of the user.

5 Data Augmentation

Learning reciprocal adaptation requires accurate data from both interlocutors. Nonetheless, we have a limited amount of clean and accurate conversation data (i.e., face-to-face data) of both interactants. This limitation led us to propose a data augmentation technique that learns from both interlocutors. During the training phase, for each batch, we randomly assign the interlocutor identity (either U1 or U2) that will be played by the agent to one of the interlocutors. By doing so, the model learns to predict the behaviors of this interlocutor. Then, the interlocutor's identity is constantly alternated and randomly reassigned to the agent. The employment of this technique allows the model to learn to predict equally the behaviors of both participants and to focus on modeling the interaction between the two rather than the specific characteristics of a single person.

At the inference stage, the agent will play the role of a single interlocutor (U1 or U2), and the user will be the other interlocutor (U2 or U1, respectively). More specifically, the identities of A and U will be assigned to the agent and user respectively.

6 Self-Attention Pruning

We model reciprocal adaptation by capturing the interpersonal relationship and multimodal information. Interpersonal behavior coherence and synchrony are learned by extracting key features from multimodal information. Relevant features are selected using the attention mechanism. We employ self-attention (multi-head attention of the Transformers [13]) with all interlocutors' visual and acoustic modalities (X^A_{speech}, X^A_{face}, X^U_{speech}, X^U_{face}) as its input. Key information is captured within the self-attention layer. Attention heads, within the multi-head attention (MHA), may contain redundant information causing the model to overfit. We solve this overfitting problem by applying pruning. With pruning, repetitive heads are dropped out rendering only dissimilar heads encoded with unique information. Another advantage of using pruning is that it increases the inference speed. We learn to choose which head(s) contain meaningful information for each specific frame via a custom pruning mask instead of pruning a given percentage of less significant neurons or connections. Via the custom pruning mask, the pruned attention heads vary for each prediction. Therefore, using our pruning technique, our model accesses unique and relevant information for each prediction.

7 Autoregressive Adaptive Online Prediction

Generating continuous behavior is essential to render natural human-like agent behavior. Adaptive online prediction is applied during the inference phase keeping the past information within the LSTM memory cells. In addition, new predictions are computed in an autoregressive fashion. Predictions made during previous time steps are fed back as the input for the new predictions (for the next time step).

7.1 Result and Discussion

To evaluate the performance of our model, we assess our ASAP model objectively and subjectively against the following baseline models:

- IL-LSTM [14]: modeling of the interpersonal relationship based only on the visual modality (facial gestures) of both the agent and human user;
- Sym-IL-LSTM [15]: modeling of the interpersonal relationship based on multi-modal features (speech and facial gestures) of both the agent and human user while assuring motion continuity.

8 Objective Evaluation

For the objective evaluation, we use the measures of RMSE (point-to-point measure), KS test (probability distribution similarity between our predictions and ground truth (i.e., real interaction)), and DTW (resemblance between our predictions and ground truth (i.e., real interaction)) assessing them against two features sets.

The two features sets are as follows.

- Features set 1: only visual features (eye movement, head rotation, and AU12 intensity and activation) of both interlocutors along with conversational state inputted to predict visual features of the agent at 5fps;
- Features set 2: visual and audio features (eye movement, head rotation, upper face AUs and AU12 intensities, fundamental frequency, loudness, voicing probability, and 13 MFCCs) of both interlocutors to predict the visual features (including upper face AUs) of the agent at 25fps.

In Table 3, we evaluated the three models quantitatively by computing the RMSE and the KS two-sample test. Both measures compare the average score of the output features: features set 1 computes the average of six output feature scores (2 eye angles, 3 head rotations, and AU12 intensity), and features set 2 computes the average of 12 output feature scores (2 eye angles, 3 head rotations, and the intensities of 6 upper face AUs and AU12). We can observe that for both features sets, ASAP performs better than the baseline models in terms of both RMSE and KS test scores.

We also compute the DTW to assess the resemblance between our agent-user interaction $\hat{Y}^A(t)\&Y^U(t)$ and the ground truth interaction (real human–human interaction) $Y^A(t)\&Y^U(t)$. The closer the DTW distance, the more the two signals $Y^A(t)$ and $Y^U(t)$ are similar. If the model's DTW distance $\hat{Y}^A(t)\&Y^U(t)$ is close to that of the ground truth interaction $Y^A(t)\&Y^U(t)$, it signifies that the model was able to produce adaptive agent behaviors that resemble real human–human interactions. In Table 4, we report the DTW distance for the smile signal AU12. We can note that our ASAP performs the best among the baseline models as its DTW distance is the closest one to the ground truth DTW for both features sets.

Table 3 Average RMSE and KS test results in [6]

Methods	RMSE	KS test	
Features set 1	IL-LSTM	0.172	0.298
	sym-IL-LSTM	0.171	0.293
	ASAP (ours)	**0.131**	**0.115**
Features set 2	IL-LSTM	0.444	0.559
	sym-IL-LSTM	0.374	0.415
	ASAP (ours)	**0.239**	**0.301**

Table 4 DTW of the smile signal AU12 in [6]

Features set	Method	DTW $Y^A(t)kY^u\{t)$ (Ground truth)	DTW $Y^A(t)kY^u(t)$
Features set 1	IL-LSTM	21.7	27.3
	sym-IL-LSTM		27.2
	ASAP (ours)		**26.9**
Features set 2	IL-LSTM	1317.5	1562.7
	sym-IL-LSTM		257.5
	ASAP (ours)		**1399.3**

9 Subjective Evaluation

Objective evaluation is not sufficient to fully assess the agent's behavior generation quality. To complement the objective evaluation, we perform user perceptive study. We show participants video clips (20 video clips of 7s) of our agent with the generated behavior interacting with a human interlocutor, as shown in Fig. 7.

The participants were then asked to score the interacting agent using a Likert scale of 5 points (1: strongly disagree, 2: disagree, 3: neutral, 4: agree, and 5: strongly agree) along 4 measurement constructs of behavior naturalness, behavior human-likeliness, interaction synchrony, and engagement.

For the analysis, participants' responses were grouped according to their corresponding construct (behavior naturalness, behavior human-likeliness, synchrony, and engagement). We compared our ASAP model against the two baseline models (IL-LSTM and sym-IL-LSTM) and the ground truth interaction simulated on a virtual agent (GT). A visualization of the distribution of each construct for the 4 evaluation conditions (GT, IL-LSTM, sym-IL-LSTM, and ASAP) can be seen in Fig. 8, and the median values are reported in Table 5.

Looking at the subjective results, we can remark that the condition GT receives the highest values for all four constructs. Comparing the three models, we can note that the scores improve in order of IL-LSTM, sym-IL-LSTM, and ASAP (increasing order) for all constructs. A rise in quality can be noticed for the behavior naturalness and human-likeliness constructs between IL-LSTM and the other two computational models (sym-IL-LSTM and our ASAP model). We assume that the use of adaptive online prediction (employed in sym-IL-LSTM and ASAP) instead of sliding window prediction (employed in IL-LSTM) resulted in this rise in the perception of the agent's naturalness and human-likeliness. We can also verify the impact of modeling

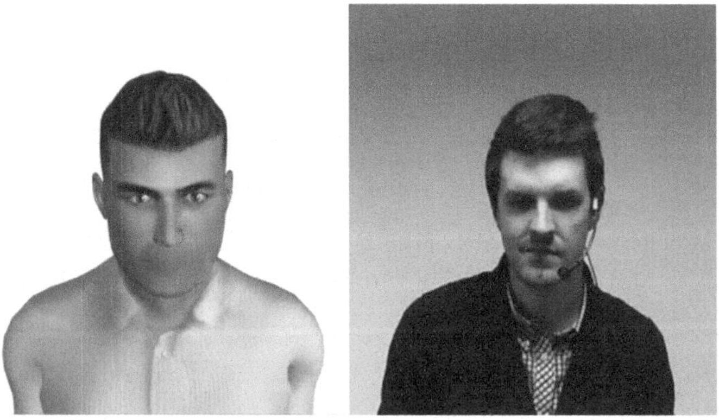

Fig. 7 User perception study video clip example of an interaction between a virtual agent (left) and its human interlocutor (right) in [6]

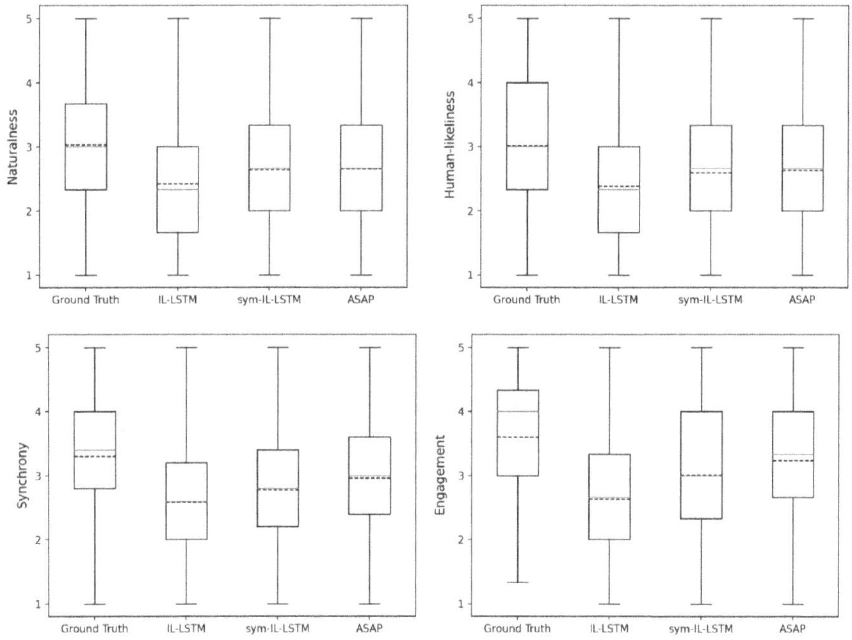

Fig. 8 Distribution of behavior naturalness (upper left), human-likeliness (upper right), synchrony (lower left), and engagement (lower right) in [6]. The median is represented by the orange line and the mean is represented by the green dashed line

Table 5 Median and mean values (median/mean) of naturalness, human-likeliness, synchrony, and engagement in [6]

Methods	Naturalness	Human-likeliness	Synchrony	Engagement
GT	3.00/3.03	3.00/3.02	3.40/3.30	4.00/3.60
IL-LSTM	2.33/2.42	2.33/2.38	2.60/2.59	2.67/2.63
sym-IL-LSTM	2.67/2.63	2.67/2.59	2.80/2.78	3.00/3.01
ASAP (ours)	**2.67/2.66**	**2.67/2.63**	**3.00/2.97**	**3.33/3.24**

reciprocal adaptation via the quality performance of ASAP. ASAP was perceived to be more in sync and engaged with its interlocutor than the other two baseline models.

Via our objective and subjective evaluation results, which are in line with each other, we can check that our ASAP model outperforms the baseline models of IL-LSTM and sym-IL-LSTM along the four constructs (naturalness, human-likeliness, synchrony, and engagement). Being the most similar one to the ground truth (i.e., real human–human interaction) both quantitatively and qualitatively, with ASAP we show how the endowment of reciprocal adaptation capability can make virtual agents behave more socially and engaged as both speaker and listener.

10 Real-Time Adaptive Virtual Agent System for Cognitive Behavioral Therapy

Virtual agents have shown their usefulness in providing medical care [16, 17], especially for Cognitive Behavior Therapy (CBT). We seek to see if a virtual agent with reciprocal adaptation capability can improve the interaction itself, more precisely the user experience (i.e., perception of the agent), and at the same time the effect of CBT.

We start by designing an adaptive virtual agent system, IAVA system [9] that provides real-time human–agent interaction. The system is able to adapt its behavior to its interacting user, generating expressive and adaptive agent behavior (i.e., facial expressions and head/gaze movements). It displays continuous agent movements at the frame level enabling real-time rendering. Within the system, the ASAP model [6] and a BERT-based language model for CBT are integrated to provide adaptive behavior and coherent verbal context to the user.

To fully assess our adaptive CBT agent, we check how human interactants perceive adaptive agents in terms of naturalness, human-likeliness, interaction synchrony, engagement, and rapport for the user experience. For the CBT effectiveness, questionnaires from the psychology field such as State-Trait Anxiety Inventory, Kessler Psychological Distress Scale (K6), Cognitive Change-Immediate Scale (CC), and self-reported mood are used.

10.1 Real-Time Adaptive Virtual Agent System Development

For the development of a real-time adaptive virtual agent, several functionalities must be assured. The agent must perceive the user's behavior and also its own behavior, generate expressive and adaptive behavior, manage its dialog, and render its behavior.

The IAVA system perceives the user's behavior (speech and gesture) via open-source tools (i.e., Google ASR for speech content, openSMILE for speech prosody, and OpenFace for user's facial gestures). As the agent needs to behave depending not only on its user's behavior but also on its own prior behavior, the agent remembers its previously generated behaviors within its internal memory. The perceived behavior of both the human user and the agent is fed to the ASAP model for the generation of expressive and adaptive agent behavior. The generated behavior is rendered and displayed at the frame-level (i.e., 25 fps) using the Greta platform [18].

Alongside the frame-level behavior visualization, the agent also manages its speech (i.e., dialog). The conversational flow, or the turn-taking present between interlocutors, is controlled depending on the speech content and speech acoustic features. The system decides, depending on the user's utterance, whether it should take the next speech turn or leave the user to continue talking. In addition, the next agent's speech content also varies taking into account the user's saying. For the selection of the agent's speech, a BERT-based language model, the automatic thought classifier [8], is used. It classifies the user's utterance identifying whether it is an automatic thought or not. Depending on the state of being an automatic thought, the next CBT-related agent speech is rendered via the CereProc speech synthesizer.

10.2 Experimental Setting

The evaluation of our adaptive virtual agent system for CBT was tested with a sample size of 60 French-speaking participants (confidence level of 90 with a margin of error of 10 for the French population with a higher education degree). For this study, we set the inclusion criteria of French-speaking, 18 years or older, and no vision or hearing impairments.

To assess the impact of having an expressive and adaptive agent (i.e., reciprocally adaptive), condition RA, we compared our agent with an agent that is solely expressive (i.e., showing mismatched movements), condition MM, and a static agent (i.e., in a still position with only lip-sync), condition SP. Each of the three experimental conditions (RA, MM, and SP) had 20 participants.

10.3 Result and Discussion

To investigate the impact of endowing adaptive capability to the agent, condition RA, we focus on evaluating the effect that our agent has on the perception of the agent and the effectiveness of CBT (user mood and state change) by comparing it against our other experimental conditions MM and SP.

We start by studying the perception of the agent felt by participants (perception of the agent's behavior) along 5 factors: naturalness, human-likeliness, synchrony, engagement, and rapport.

Via the results presented in Fig. 9. and Table 6, we can note that the agent displaying reciprocally adaptive behavior (RA condition) is perceived to be the most natural, human-like, in sync, engaged, and to have a rapport with the participant compared to the other two agents (MM and SP conditions). While it is expected for an adaptive agent to be perceived more positively than an agent that shows random behavior (MM) or a static agent (SP), it is interesting to see that an agent with no motion (SP) is better perceived than an expressive agent with random and unsynced behaviors (MM). The display of random behavior seems to hinder the impression of the agent. This means that it is better to remain still than to show non-adaptive behavior. Thus, for an agent to be well perceived it is essential to produce behaviors that consider the interlocutor.

Concerning the effect each condition has on CBT, we look at the change the agent has on the user's mood, anxiety state change, psychological distress level change, and cognitive change via self-reported mood, State-Trait Anxiety Inventory, Kessler

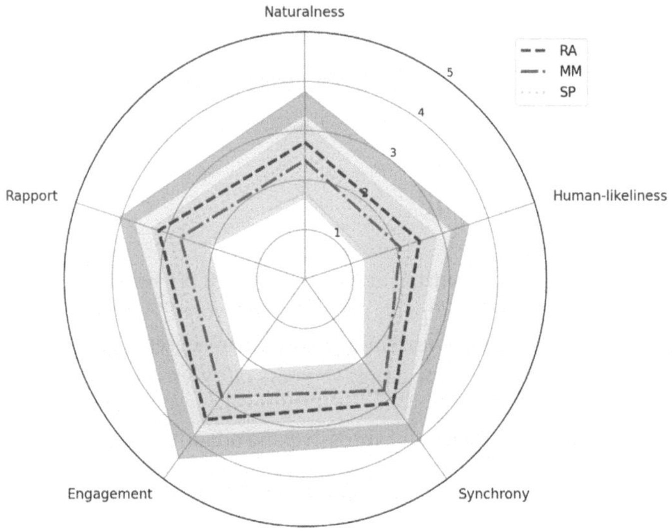

Fig. 9 Perception of the agent's behavior along naturalness, human-likeliness, synchrony, engagement, and rapport in [8]. The central line in bold represents the mean value of each condition (RA, MM, and SP) and the colored-filled contour represents the standard deviation of each condition

Table 6 Mean and standard deviation of agent behavior perception factors for the conditions of RA, MM, and SP in [8]

Factor	RA		MM		SP	
	Mean	SD	Mean	SD	Mean	SD
Naturalness	2.77	1.030	2.40	0.762	2.55	0.728
Human-likeliness	2.50	1.070	2.08	0.779	2.30	0.871
Synchrony	3.11	0.941	2.79	0.706	2.86	0.732
Engagement	3.52	0.964	2.95	0.678	3.23	0.659
Rapport	3.18	0.860	2.72	0.620	2.95	0.743

Factor	Between RA-MM		Between RA-SP	
	Cohen's d	*P*-value	Cohen's d	*P*-value
Naturalness	1.28	0.210	0.767	0.448
Human-likeliness	1.41	0.169	0.647	0.522
Synchrony	1.22	0.232	0.938	0.355
Engagement	2.15	0.039	1.085	0.286
Rapport	1.97	0.057	0.935	0.356

Significance difference between the condition pairs (RA, MM) and (RA, SP) reported via one-sided Welch's *t*-test

Psychological Distress Scale (K6), and Cognitive Change-Immediate Scale (CC), respectively. The results of each

CBT measure are reported in Table 7.

Looking at the mood change scores, we can remark on the difference that each experimental condition (RA, MM, and SP) has. An adaptive agent (RA) is better at ameliorating the participants' mood during the CBT session compared to when the agent remains in a constant position (SP). Nevertheless, a non-adaptive agent (MM) may trigger stronger changes. In mood scores. The presence of the agent's movement may have helped the improvement of participants' mood by easing the participants' feelings via the production of expressive visual feedback independent of the presence of adaptation.

The anxiety level change is reported via STAI-State inventory. We note differences in the anxiety change between the three experimental conditions (RA, MM, and SP). Reciprocally adaptive agent (RA) improves the anxiety state of the participants during the CBT session while agents without motion (SP) or random motions (MM) may even worsen the anxiety level of the participants.

Psychological distress level, obtained with the K6 scale, seems to improve when the agent is expressive (RA and MM) regardless of whether the expressive behavior is interlocutor-adaptive or not. The expressivity present within the agents may allow participants to think that the agent is physically present before them making them feel psychologically relieved to interact with the agent and fully benefit from the interaction of the CBT treatment.

Along with the positive influence of exhibiting expressive behavior, we can also assume that the display of adaptive behaviors (RA) can further lessen the stress level

Table 7 Mean and standard deviation of user mood and state measures for the conditions of RA, MM, and SP in [8]

Measure	RA		MM		SP	
	Mean	SD	Mean	SD	Mean	SD
Mood change score	0.376	0.251	0.483	0.313	0.246	0.440
ΔSTAI-State	1.40	7.63	− 0.50	4.67	− 1.20	6.49
ΔK6	1.95	3.39	0.85	2.74	− 0.10	2.43
CC	11.8	7.30	10.2	6.58	11.0	5.20

Measure	Between RA-MM		Between RA-SP	
	Cohen's d	*P*-value	Cohen's d	*P*-value
Mood change score	− 1.192	0.241	1.149	0.260
ΔSTAI-State	0.949	0.350	1.161	0.253
ΔK6	1.128	0.267	2.197	0.035
CC	0.705	0.485	0.374	0.711

Significance difference between the condition pairs (RA, MM) and (RA, SP) reported via one-sided Welch's t-test than showing solely expressive behaviors (MM). Nevertheless, when interacting with an agent in a fixed position (SP), the participants may become more stressed.

Via this study, we validated the impact of an agent showing adaptive behavior. The endowment of reciprocal adaptation capacity enables agents to be perceived positively. The impression of agents becomes similar to that of a real human in terms of being natural, human-like, in sync, engaged, and building a rapport. For the effectiveness of CBT, we checked that adaptive agents (RA) render higher CBT effects than other agents that are static (SP) or simply expressive with no adaptation (MM).

We also observed an intriguing result in which a non-expressive (SP) agent was perceived better than a non-adaptive but still expressive agent (MM). Thus, it is better to not show any behavior than to simply express via the exhibition of random behavior that does not consider the interlocutor. Nevertheless, displaying random expressive behavior can still be useful in the fields of medical and psychological healthcare. Our results show that the sole expression can heighten the CBT effects as the agent's expressivity may intensify the user's feeling of its physical presence resulting in a better CBT treatment.

Adaptive agents are thus not only beneficial in enhancing the user experience but also in healthcare applications.

11 Conclusion

Adaptation is an essential communication skill. For virtual agents to interact with human users, they also need to know how to adapt to their interlocutors. Via this work, we looked into how we can evaluate adaptation, generate adaptive behavior from multimodal interaction data, and develop a real-time adaptive virtual agent system that can be applied to CBT. Via our study, we showed that agents with adaptation capability can improve the user experience by providing a positive agent impression in terms of naturalness, human-likeliness, synchrony, engagement, and rapport. Furthermore, employing them for the delivery of CBT can enhance the effect of CBT notably the users' moods and states (anxiety, psychological distress, and cognitive).

Acknowledgements Funding was provided by ANR-JST-CREST TAPAS [grant number ANR-19-JSTS-0001] project.

This chapter is an extension of the PhD thesis of the first author which was done at ISIR, Sorbonne University.

References

1. W.S. Condon, W.D. Ogston, A segmentation of behavior. J. Psychiatr. Res., pp. 221–35, (1967)

2. J.K. Burgoon, L.A. Stern, L. Dillman, Interpersonal adaptation: dyadic interaction patterns. Cambridge University Press, (1995)
3. F.J. Bernieri, R. Rosenthal, Interpersonal coordination: behavior matching and interactional synchrony. Stud. Emot. Soc. Interact. Fundam. Nonverbal Behav. 401–32. (1991)
4. T.L. Chartrand, J.L. Lakin, The antecedents and consequences of human behavioral mimicry. Ann. Rev. Psychol. 285–308. (2013)
5. J. Woo, C. Pelachaud, C. Achard, *Reciprocal adaptation measures for human-agent interaction evaluation.* In Proceedings of the 15th International Conference on Agents and Artificial Intelligence, (2023)
6. J. Woo, C. Pelachaud, C. Achard, *ASAP: endowing adaptation capability to agent in human-agent interaction.* In Proceedings of the 28th International Conference on Intelligent User Interfaces (IUI '23), (2023), pp. 464–475
7. J. Woo, M. Fares, C. Pelachaud, C. Achard, AMII: Adaptive Multimodal Inter-personal and Intra-personal Model for Adapted Behavior Synthesis. (2023) arXivpreprintarXiv:2305.11310
8. J. Woo, K. Shidara, C. Achard, H. Tanaka, S. Nakamura, C. Pelachaud, Adaptive virtual agent: Design and evaluation for real-time human-agent interaction. Int. J. Human Comput. Stud. 103321, (2024)
9. J. Woo, M. Grimaldi, C. Pelachaud, C. Achard, *IAVA: Interactive and Adaptive Virtual Agent.* In Proceedings of the 23rd ACM International Conference on Intelligent Virtual Agents. (2023), pp 1–8
10. A. Cafaro, J. Wagner, T. Baur, S. Dermouche, M. Torres Torres, C. Pelachaud, E. André, M. Valstar, *The NoXi database: multimodal recordings of mediated novice-expert interactions.* In Proceedings of the 19th ACM International Conference on Multimodal Interaction. (2017), pp. 350–359
11. P. Ekman, An argument for basic emotions. Cogn. Emot. 169–200, (1992)
12. T.L. Chartrand, J.A. Bargh, The chameleon effect: The perception–behavior link and social interaction. J. Pers. Soc. Psychol. 893 (1999)
13. A. Vaswani, Attention is all you need. Adv. Neural Inform. Process. Syst., (2017)
14. S. Dermouche, C. Pelachaud, *Generative model of agent's behaviors in human-agent interaction.* In 2019 International Conference on Multimodal Interaction. (2019), pp 375–384
15. J. Woo, C. Pelachaud, C. Achard, Creating an interactive human/agent loop using multimodal recurrent neural networks. In WACAI 2021, (2021)
16. L. Ring, T. Bickmore, P. Pedrelli, *An affectively aware virtual therapist for depression counseling.* In ACM SIGCHI Conference on Human Factors in Computing Systems (CHI) workshop on Computing and Mental Health, (2016), pp. 01951–12
17. K. Shidara, H. Tanaka, H. Adachi, D. Kanayama, Y. Sakagami, T. Kudo, S. Nakamura, Automatic thoughts and facial expressions in cognitive restructuring with virtual agents. Front. Comput. Sci., 762424, (2022)
18. R. Niewiadomski, E. Bevacqua, M. Mancini, C. Pelachaud, *Greta: an interactive expressive ECA system*, In Proceedings of The 8th International Conference on Autonomous Agents and Multiagent Systems, (2009), pp. 1399–1400

Virtual Reality and Augmented Reality

Yuichiro Fujimoto

Abstract Public speaking skills, the ability to address large audiences and interact with individuals, are crucial in social life. This chapter presents two studies on applying virtual reality (VR) technologies to public speaking training and support. The first study investigates the use of VR for reflection on public speaking training. Commonly, individuals record and review their presentations to identify areas for improvement. However, reviewing one's own videos can cause discomfort and hinder objective self-assessment. To address this issue, the study confirmed the effectiveness of employing an avatar with a different appearance and using VR to review presentations from the audience's perspective [38]. The second study examines the provision of real-time feedback in a VR environment. In VR, comprehensive data, including body movements, gaze, speech, and slide manipulation, can be utilized to detect issues and provide immediate feedback. However, due to the cognitive demands of the presentation, users may not always accept feedback. To alleviate this problem, the possibility of estimating feedback timing that is inappropriate for the user from observable information was investigated [8].

1 Background and Overview

Public speaking can instill fear in speakers regardless of their experience level. Individuals with conditions like autism spectrum disorder (ASD) often exhibit heightened anxiety. Furthermore, statistics show that about 77% of the general population experiences a fear of public speaking, making it the most prevalent social fear [9, 32]. This fear and anxiety can negatively impact the quality of a presentation by affecting a speaker's cognitive resources, eye movements, body posture, and hand gestures. Generally, people engage in repeated practice sessions to manage their internal state.[1]

[1] https://human-gc.jp/english/

Y. Fujimoto (✉)
Ryukoku University, Kyoto, Japan
e-mail: yfujimoto@rins.ryukoku.ac.jp

S. Nakamura (ed.), *Multimodal Interaction Technologies for Training Affective Social Skills*, https://doi.org/10.1007/978-981-96-1313-7_9

And behavior before a presentation. However, while rehearsing in a similar environment to the actual presentation is ideal, it is often costly. Therefore, a more accessible method is needed.

Recently, various presentation training programs utilizing virtual reality (VR) technology have emerged, allowing for the creation of realistic scenarios at a lower cost using 3D models in a virtual setting [25, 31]. VR systems enable users to refine their presentation skills extensively without the concern of receiving immediate feedback from others [16, 20]. Many VR-based training systems monitor and assess the presenter's performance during practice, offering feedback either during or after the session. These systems have been shown to effectively enhance presentation skills.

We have conducted two studies that utilize the intrinsic characteristics of VR more effectively and explore new possibilities for applying them to public speaking training and support.

The first study explores the application of VR in reflecting on public speaking training. A common practice for preparing presentations that involve speaking in front of an audience and using slides is to record oneself and review the footage to identify areas for improvement. However, watching one's own video can induce discomfort, and maintaining objectivity in self-assessment is often challenging. To address this issue, the study examined the effectiveness of using avatars that look different from oneself and incorporating VR to change perspectives, allowing for reflection on one's presentation from the audience's viewpoint.

The second study focuses on real-time feedback in VR at appropriate moments. In a VR environment, various data such as body movements, gaze information, speech, and slide manipulation are available, enabling the automatic detection of issues and providing immediate feedback to the user. However, since giving a presentation is a cognitively demanding task, users may not always be able to accept feedback at all times. To mitigate this issue, the study proposed a mechanism to estimate the most suitable timing for feedback for the user and confirmed its effectiveness.

2 VR Reflection for Public Speaking Training

2.1 Overview

This research aimed to enhance speakers' self-awareness through self-reflection [38]. Video reflection is a well-established pedagogical tool for basic public speaking training, allowing for the recording and later analysis of both verbal and nonverbal aspects of speech performance. This technique helps individuals improve their skill acquisition, speech content, objective test performance, and recall of the actual speech [4]. However, individuals with public speaking anxiety often have low self-esteem and confidence, making them more likely to avoid video feedback due to a reluctance to watch their own performance [21].

To address this challenge, this study explored a straightforward VR-based reflection system. Utilizing VR and a head-mounted display (HMD), the system allows presenters to view their behavior from a third-person perspective within a 3D VR environment. This can enhance subjective ratings of an observer-like perspective during recall [18] and provide a broader field of view (FOV) compared to video, potentially leading to improved self-reflection. A 3D human model serves as the presenter's avatar, focusing solely on elements that evaluate the quality of the presentation without affecting the presenter's mood in the VR space. This paper details an experimental study using this VR-based reflection system, examining which populations could benefit the most and evaluating the impact of factors like the avatar and other HMD-based VR elements on the effectiveness of reflection.

The requirements for effective self-reflection in this context are: (R1) Awareness of one's problems during a presentation, (R2) Understanding one's visibility to others without cognitive bias, and (R3) Avoiding excessive self-focused attention and negative emotions.

To achieve all of these requirements, idea (A) a unique VR characteristic in which information can be confirmed by placing one's body in a state close to the real world (i.e., in a 3D space), and idea (B) the characteristics that enable the selective display of only the necessary information were used in this study.

2.1.1 Reflections from a Third-Person Perspective

In the real world, people adjust their perceived visual information based on their body, head, and eye gaze positions. They can sense their posture and location even with their eyes closed, maintaining consistency between perceived and physical positions. However, in VR, when a human-shaped 3D avatar is displayed in front of a presenter, its position might not align with the presenter's perceived position. This discrepancy can make the avatar seem like another person, though it represents the past self [22]. Objectively evaluating others tends to be more accurate than self-evaluation [1].

Additionally, a wider FOV in VR can enhance spatial awareness and memory of peripheral information, making it similar to a real observer's experience [13]. Thus, applying idea (A) in HMD-based VR is expected to yield similar effects.

2.1.2 Appearance Factor

Nonverbal communication plays a crucial role in public speaking, encompassing posture, gestures, facial expressions, gaze patterns, and acoustic characteristics [3, 28]. Directly viewing oneself on video can cause psychological resistance [21].

In this study, we categorized appearance factors based on their impact on presentation quality and mood interference, visualizing only the necessary information. Our policy aimed to exclude unique appearance details, although altering one's physical appearance while maintaining controllable features during the presentation proved challenging, with a few technical exceptions. The elements that were employed in this study are Position, Body Posture, Face Direction, Hand/Arm Movement, and Voice. On the other hand, we did not use eye gaze, personal facial appearance, personal body form, and clothing.

2.2 System Implementation

The experimental system's general architecture is proposed in [14]. It operates in two modes: presentation and playback. In presentation mode, users can practice their presentations in a virtual environment that simulates a real setting. The system records the user's behaviors, including speech and body movements, during the presentation. After processing the user's behavior, the system creates a sequential motion with a virtual avatar. When the system works in the playback mode, users can watch the VR presentation recording using the HMD or a normal PC monitor.

2.2.1 Hardware

The system comprises a PC, an HTC VIVE Pro Eye HMD (Dual OLED, 1440 × 1600 pixels per eye) with two base stations for tracking, a Microsoft Azure Kinect depth camera for body measurement, a Panasonic RP-HX350 stereo microphone, and a VIVE controller for slide control. All components run in Unity on a single PC (CPU: Core i7-5930K, 3.50GHz, RAM: 16GB, OS: Windows 10 Enterprise). Figure 1 shows the setup location of each component.

2.2.2 Presentation Mode

The proposed system allows presenters to deliver presentations in a VR environment, similar to previous studies. A VR environment was constructed to imitate a small office meeting room. In this virtual space, the presenter stands in front of a projector screen in a $4 \times 6\ m^2$ conference room and can walk around occasionally. Three virtual audience members are seated in front, nodding and taking notes on their computers intermittently. The screen displays the presentation slides, and the presenter can use the VIVE controller to navigate between slides. In this environment, presenters can repeatedly practice their presentations. The information described below is recorded during the presentation.

2.2.3 Playback Mode

This mode is the main function of this study. The user, wearing the HMD, can observe the information recorded in presentation mode from an observer's perspective (Fig. 2). The user takes a seat as an audience member, and the viewpoint changes

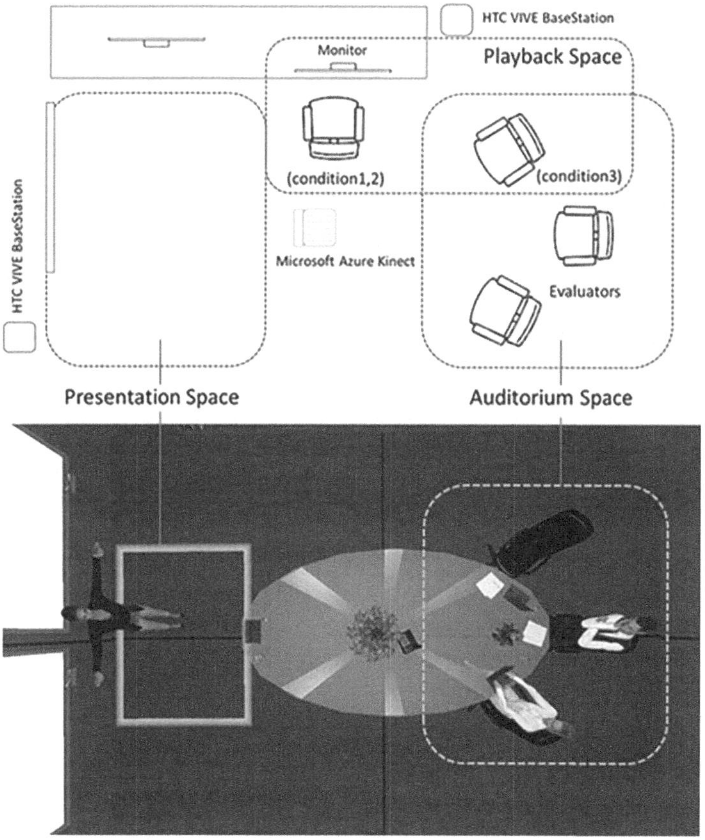

Fig. 1 System setting. Top: The setting in the real environment. Bottom: The corresponding VR environment in the playback mode

with their head movements. An avatar was prepared for each gender. The height of the avatars was adjusted to match the participant's height measured using Azure Kinect in the presentation phase. The information recorded, the recording method in the presentation mode, and how to use the recorded information in the playback mode are described in the following sections.

Position and Posture: The posture was considered as a group of positions of 32 joints of the human body and was recorded by Azure Kinect as 3D positions and postures at 30 frames per second. The 3D position of the spine was used as the human location in the environment.

Hand/Arm Movement: The arm postures were also recorded using Azure Kinect. The arm contains four joint points in each posture. Owing to accuracy issues, the hand states were defined and recorded as either open or closed.

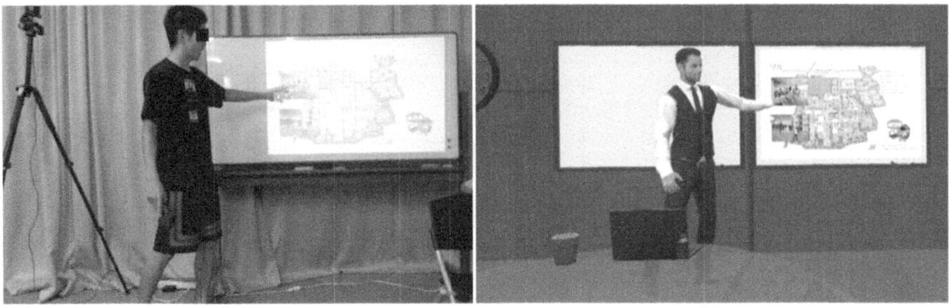

(a) (b)

Fig. 2 Example of the system view. **a** Recorded user in the presentation mode. **b** Corresponding avatar in the playback mode

Voice: The voice was saved in a stereo form since it was the user's original voice. By combining the voice with the 3D standing position, a stereo sound that was generated from the spatially correct sound source position was presented to the user.

Slide Switching Timing: The slide switch timing was also recorded so that the slides can be viewed during the playback.

2.3 Evaluation

2.3.1 Method

The experiment evaluated the effectiveness of avatars and HMD-based VR for reflection, focusing on individual differences. Participants first gave a presentation using predefined slides, which was recorded by the system. They then reviewed their presentations in VR to identify improvements before giving a second presentation. Effectiveness was measured by changes in self-reported anxiety, self-evaluations before and after playback, and differences in self-evaluations or experimenter evaluations between the two presentations.

2.3.2 Participants

For this investigation, 24 graduate students (13 males, 11 females, aged 22–42 years, M = 27.04, SD = 4.30), all non-native English speakers, from a local university were recruited via email. The Personal Report of Confidence as a Speaker (PRCS) score assessed their fear of public speaking before the experiment. Participants were divided into three groups based on PRCS scores to ensure an equal distribution of self-confidence.

Each participant received a 2,000 JPY honorarium for the two-hour experiment. Additionally, three evaluators (graduate students in information science, one male and two females) were hired to assess the presentation quality.

2.3.3 Experimental Condition

To evaluate the impact of the avatar and other parts in HMD-based VR in reflection, three conditions were set in the experiment, and the experiment was conducted as a between-subjects experiment. The participants were all asked to present without wearing HMD to make sure they gave the presentation in the same environment under all conditions. Figure 3 provide an overview of these conditions.

Condition 1: Video + PC Monitor

This setup replicated a typical individual public speaking training method where participants reviewed a video recorded by a Logitech C920 PRO HD Webcam on a standard PC monitor (Resolution: 1920 × 1200 pixels). Participants listened to the audio through headphones connected to the monitor. They used general software (Microsoft Movies & TV) to watch the videos and could replay the footage as needed using a mouse.

Condition 2: 3D Avatar + PC Monitor

In this condition, participants viewed the VR environment and 3D avatar videos on a PC monitor, reconstructed from the recorded data as described in Sect. 2.2.3. The viewpoint was aligned with the camera position to closely match condition 1, allowing similar adjustments as with regular video. The 3D avatar's motions were defined by the 3D joint positions captured by Kinect at 30 fps, mimicking the participants' movements during the presentation. The interface for controlling the video playback was identical to that in condition 1.

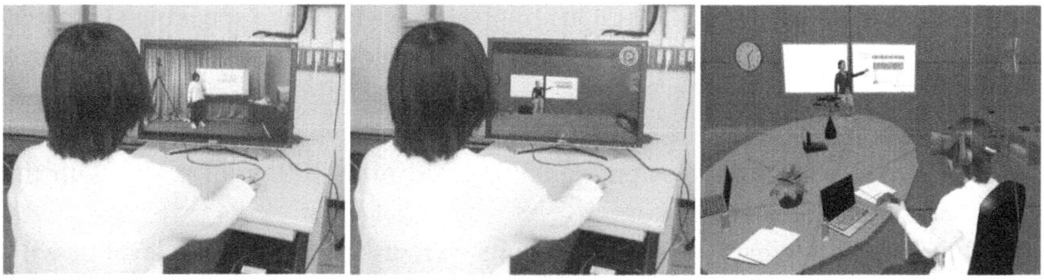

(a) (b) (c)

Fig. 3 Experimental conditions for checking participants' own presentation: **a** Condition 1: Recorded video on a PC monitor. **b** Condition 2: Avatar constructed from the recorded information on the PC monitor. **c** Condition 3: Avatar constructed from the recorded information with a head-mounted display

Condition 3: 3D Avatar + HMD

Similar to condition 2, condition 3 also utilized a 3D avatar, but instead of a PC monitor, an HMD was used as the display device. The participant was initially seated, as depicted in Fig. 1, representing the position of an audience member in the virtual environment. With the HMD, the participant's viewpoint changes based on their position and orientation, allowing them to observe their own presentation from various angles and perspectives.

2.3.4 Outcome Measurements

One of the aims of this experiment is to explore the benefits for presenters with different personality traits from the reflection.

The benefits of a reflection method for public speaking are considered in mainly three parts: changes in anxiety for public speaking, changes in subjective impression, and improvement of public speaking skills. The attention pattern in the playback and the willingness to use this system were also measured as the supplement for the performance of the method since the attention part could lead to the result of reflection and the willingness will lead to the dropout rate of the training.

The questionnaires used for this experiment are as follows. By using these questionnaires, the personal characteristics of the presenter and training indicators of the training method were measured.

Anxiety (Anx) To measure anxiety changes in public speaking, the PRCS [12, 15] was used. This 12-item questionnaire evaluates fear on a scale of 1–10.

Presentation quality by self (SQu) Subjective impressions of presentation performance were measured using the public speaking competence rubric (PSCR) score from [29], which includes 11 questions focusing on content, voice, and body movement for self-assessment. Four questions related to preparation and organization were excluded since the material was pre-prepared. Additionally, a 100-point scale was used to rate the overall impression.

Presentation quality by others (OQu) Improvement in public speaking skills was measured using the PSCR score for assessment by evaluators. Two out of three randomly assigned evaluators were assessed immediately after the presentation. Despite being non-experts, the PSCR allows for objective and quantitative assessments [29]. An overall impression was also rated on a 100-point scale, with the average score used as an indicator.

Willingness of playback (Wil) Participants were asked to score the level of willingness to use the playback method in each condition based on a 5-point scale (1: strongly disagree, 5: strongly agree).

Presenter Characteristics

To identify the target users of a VR reflection system, this experiment considered personal confidence, self-bias, and public speaking anxiety due to their relationship with presentation performance and reflection. Although gender is not considered a factor in presentation or reflection quality, its impact on other characteristics, such as self-bias [33], and its effect on public speaking training remains controversial.

Gender: The role of gender in managing public speaking anxiety remains a topic of debate. Generally, gender differences do not have a significant impact on public speaking anxiety [11]. However, some studies have reported that gender differences can affect certain training outcomes [2].

Personal confidence for public speaking skills confidence encourages individuals to embrace challenges and reflect on their approach [34]. It remains unclear whether the observer perspective provided by our VR reflection method helps individuals with lower confidence to better focus on their presentation approach. Confidence in public speaking skills was assessed on a 5-point scale (1: very poor, 5: excellent) prior to the experiment.

Self-bias: The disparity between SQu and OQu indicates self-bias. Some individuals struggle with fair self-assessment due to biased cognition, which can lead to ineffective reflection. This paper explores how self-bias is affected by the use of avatars and VR during playback. To evaluate overall impressions of personal characteristics, a 100-point scale was used for measuring presentation-specific aspects, given that the PSCR score emphasizes individual presentation elements.

Personal anxiety for public speaking public speaking anxiety has been widely discussed in the context of public speaking training [5, 26, 30]. Typically, personal anxiety correlates with negative self-assessment according to cognitive models. However, some reports indicate that individuals with social anxiety may not underestimate their performance [24]. Therefore, personal anxiety and self-bias were considered as separate characteristics to analyze the results. Anxiety was measured using the PRCS from personal reports before the experiment, reflecting general fear.

2.3.5 Training Indicators

First, for the question of how the anxiety for public speaking was reduced, the changes after the playback and after the whole experiment were measured:

Anxiety changing(p1-pb) The Anx for Presentation 1 changing between the personal reports before and after playback.

Anxiety changing(p1-p2) The Anx changing between two presentations, indicating the anxiety reduction from the training.

For how did the playback change the subjective impression, the following indicators were measured:

Self-assessment changing(pb-p1) The Self-assessment changing is measured by PSCR score in SQu after playback. Since the Self-bias from presenter characteristics also use PSCR score in SQu before playback, so we will not analyze the relation of Self-bias and Self-assessment changing.

Bias changing (p1-pb) The self-bias changing of assessment from reflection is measured as the changes in absolute value of gaps between SQu and OQu before and after playback. Similar to Self-assessment changing, the Self-bias from presenter characteristics also use SQu before playback, so we will not analyze the relation of them.

At last, for the question of public speaking skill improvement in the whole training, both subjective and objective indicators were measured:

Subjective improvement(p2-p1) The personal feeling about the improvement in public speaking skills, measured by PSCR score changing in SQu between two presentations.

Objective improvement(p2-p1) More objective results for the presenter's improvement on public speaking skills, measured by PSCR score changing in OQu between two presentations.

2.3.6 Procedures

The process of the experiment is as follows.

Introduction and Consent: The experimenter provided each participant with an overview of the experiment and obtained their informed consent. Participants were then instructed on how to use the system for each condition. They were briefed on the presentation theme, the slides, and the content of each slide. For this experiment, 10 slides were prepared on the topic "Introduce Your University" for a five-minute presentation. This topic was selected to minimize differences in participants' prior knowledge. Participants were given 10 minutes to prepare their initial presentation. First Presentation: Participants delivered the first presentation using the prepared slides (Presentation 1) while standing in the designated presentation area, as shown in Fig. 2. They presented to three individuals: two evaluators hired according to their availability and one experimenter seated in the experimental room. This setup was intended to increase social anxiety for the presenter [26]. Primarily, evaluations from the two hired evaluators were used, but if their ratings were inconsistent, the experimenter's rating was also considered, with the average score used as the final assessment. Self-Assessment and Reflection: After Presentation 1, participants completed the PSCR to evaluate their presentation quality and the PRCS to assess their anxiety levels. The evaluators also provided ratings based on the PSCR. Participants then reviewed the recorded presentation and engaged in self-reflection. They identified areas for improvement and practiced using the playback method described in Sect. 2.2.3. Participants could view the video recording once, complete a questionnaire about the DoC for each part, and re-assess their performance with the PSCR and PRCS to note any changes in self-assessment. Participants were then given an additional 10 minutes to review specific parts, pausing each scene with a mouse (conditions 1 and 2) or a VR controller (condition 3). This phase ended once participants felt they had adequately reviewed and trained, even if the 10 minutes had elapsed. Second Presentation: Participants delivered a second 5-minute presentation on the same topic (Presentation 2), applying insights gained during the reflection phase. After this presentation, they completed the PSCR and PRCS again, and the evaluators assessed the presentation using the PSCR.

Post-Experiment Interview: Finally, a brief interview was conducted to gather participants' feedback on the experiment.

2.4 Results

Four personal characteristics: gender, personal anxiety, personal confidence, and self-bias, were mainly considered.

An analysis of independent-samples t-test was conducted for gender differences. As the result indicated, there was no significant tendency between gender and any other training indicator. In addition, there was no significant tendency between gender and other personal characteristics either.

Then an analysis of bivariate correlation was conducted for other personal characteristics (Fig. 4) and the analysis results shown in Fig. 4a indicated that there's no significant correlation among the personal characteristics.

As shown in Fig. 4b, the results of condition 3 indicated a significant correlation between personal confidence of public speaking skills and self-assessment changing(pb-p1) and objectivity changing(p1-pb), respectively, which means the participants with low personal confidence of public speaking skills could become more confident and more objective in self-assessment after VR reflection.

In Fig. 4c, the correlation between the gaps of self- and others-assessment and anxiety changing was significant in condition 3 and combination of condition 2 and condition 3, which suggested that the participants with lower self-assessment than others could reduce more anxiety in condition 2 and condition 3.

The evaluators' scores indicate that the agreement with a maximal distance of 2 ranges within 99.4 % for each of the seven aspects, which shows high overall agreement between the evaluators. However, there was no factor corrected with objective improvement in all conditions.

The Wil with the question "Would you like to use this playback method for practice?" was also considered, as it may affect long-term training. The result showed a negative correlation between the personal anxiety level and the willingness to playback for condition 2, as shown in Fig. 4d.

2.5 Discussion

The experiment results indicated that participants with low self-confidence in their public speaking skills could positively alter their subjective impressions and align them more closely with objective assessments from others after experiencing VR reflection. Individuals with low self-confidence typically avoided reviewing their own performances. One possible reason for this is that the avatar and wider field of view in condition 3 provided an objective and interactive perspective, leading to an impartial evaluation and enabling fair self-assessment. On the contrary, those

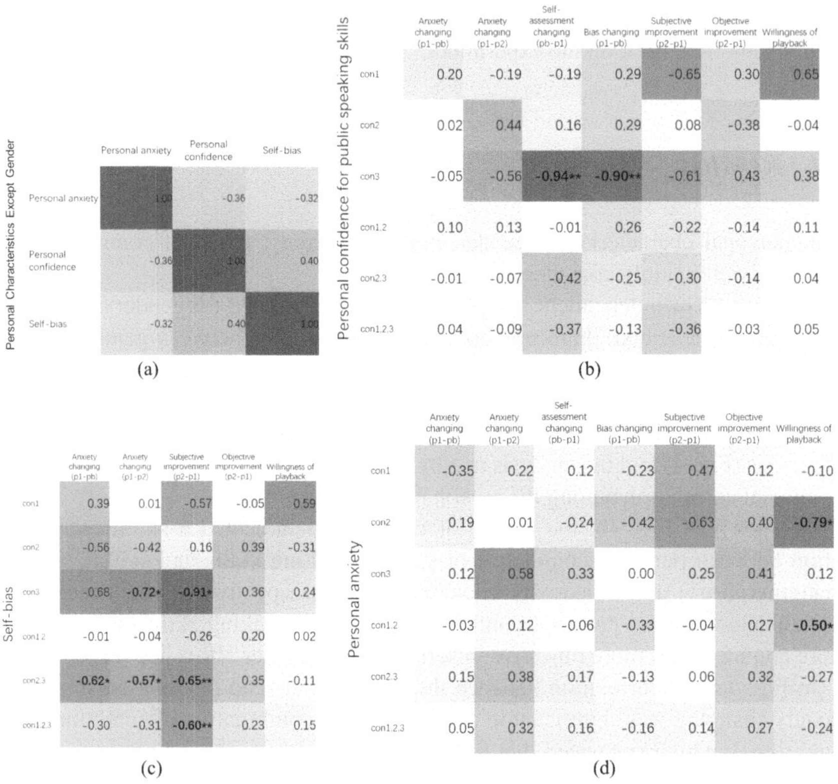

Fig. 4 Correlation: **a** among each personal characteristic except gender, **b** between personal confidence for public speaking skills and training indicators as well as Wil, **c** between self-bias and training indicators as well as Wil, **d** between personal anxiety for public speaking and training indicators as well as Wil. $**$ indicates $p < 0.01$. $*$ indicates $p < 0.05$

confident in their public speaking abilities did not harbor negative impressions of their appearance, making them less fearful and more inclined to reflect in condition 1, which offered the most factual information.

A similar perspective also proved beneficial for individuals with negative self-bias, reducing their anxiety, but they benefited more from using an avatar, according to the results. Although negative self-evaluation does not always have adverse effects, significant self-bias can highlight negative self-images in individuals. Numerous experimental studies have shown the harmful effects of negative self-image in both highly socially anxious and non-anxious participants. Individuals with self-bias tend to assess themselves more negatively compared to how they assess others, which is attributed to self-awareness. Self-awareness leads to concerns about how others perceive them, and it is linked to increased social anxiety and negative self-assessment. When people see an avatar resembling their real self, self-awareness is heightened. Therefore, it might be that using an avatar that excludes as much information about a person's unique appearance as possible can diminish self-awareness from reflection, thereby reducing anxiety. However, further evaluation of this perspective change is needed to fully understand the reason.

Some participants did note that while they recognized their weaknesses, they did not know how to improve them (e.g., "I know I should face the audience, but I cannot do this"). Alternative methods of skill acquisition should be considered.

3 Real-Time Feedback Using Proper Timing Estimation

3.1 Overview

A VR training system can generally capture head movements, controller interactions, voice, gaze data, etc. With this information, the system can potentially evaluate user performance and provide interactive feedback. For effective feedback, it is important to consider both "what" and "how" feedback is provided. This has been extensively studied (e.g., [6, 27]). This study, however, focuses on the timing ("when") of feedback delivery. Feedback can be broadly categorized into real-time feedback (concurrent feedback), which is given during the training, and summary feedback (terminal feedback), which is provided after the training or during brief breaks [23]. Summary feedback offers broad suggestions for overall performance, while real-time feedback is anticipated to be more effective for improving specific operations by addressing issues as they arise.

This research examines real-time feedback within the context of public speaking training. We considered a scenario where a trainee, wearing an HMD, delivers a presentation to a virtual audience, and the system highlights issues in the trainee's performance with corresponding icons. The advantages of real-time feedback in VR training systems have been noted [27]. However, if a significant portion of a user's cognitive resources is devoted to the ongoing task, additional real-time feedback and prompts for confirmation might disrupt the task [17] (i.e., the presentation in this study). To our knowledge, no studies have specifically investigated the negative aspects of real-time feedback and solutions within VR presentation training scenarios.

Therefore, the first research question for this study was: "To what extent does real-time feedback negatively impact presentations in VR training?" The secondary question was: "Can we estimate the timing of feedback that could negatively affect the presentation from observable information up to that point?" To address this, we developed a presentation training system using a VR-HMD to gather multimodal data (including body posture/movement, gaze, heart activity, perspiration, voice, and slide operations). Through a Wizard of Oz (WoZ) experiment with this system, we collected participants' subjective evaluations of behavioral changes and disturbances for various types of feedback. Data analysis revealed that real-time feedback occasionally had negative effects on presenters. Additionally, we found that it is possible to estimate more than half of the feedback likely to cause such negative effects from the multimodal data. These findings can guide the development of future training systems that deliver real-time feedback while avoiding inappropriate timing for the trainee [8].

3.2 Method

3.2.1 Expected Behavior of Ideal System

Figure 5 illustrates a simplified model of the proposed system's functionality. The system is designed to continuously monitor the trainee's behavior during the presentation and identify areas needing improvement (e.g., "You are gazing only on the slides instead of the audience!").

When the system detects areas requiring improvement, it assesses the trainee's acceptance to the feedback. If the trainee's acceptance is deemed low, the system will withhold feedback. Then, when the trainee is determined to have a high level of acceptance of feedback, and if the points of improvement are still evident, this feedback is presented to the trainee. We anticipate that such an approach will enhance the effectiveness of the training.

Conversely, consistently failing to present feedback when needed would be counterproductive for training. This study, however, primarily focuses on avoiding feedback delivery during moments of low acceptance, as these are likely to negatively impact the presentation.

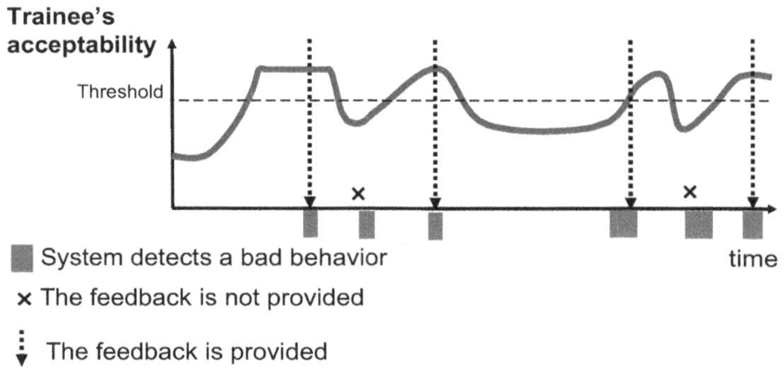

Fig. 5 Ideal system behavior to the user's acceptability

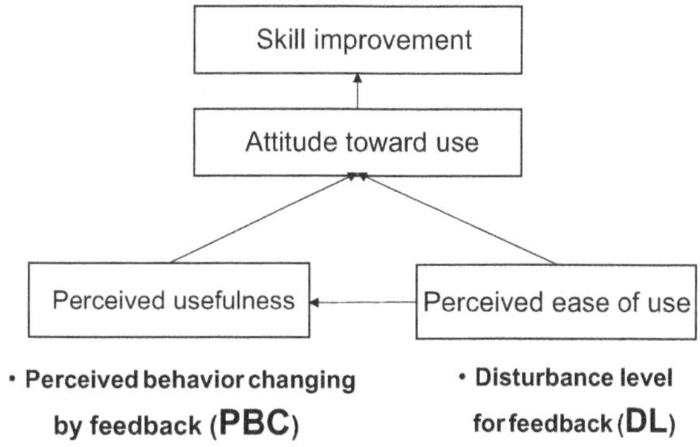

Fig. 6 Expected training effect model in real-time feedback system for public speaking. Red factors are employed in this study. Black parts come from the model in [10]

3.2.2 User's Internal Model in Training with VR System

The primary aim of the system is for trainees to develop optimal presentation skills. Mastery of many skills requires more than a single training session; ongoing practice is essential for improvement. Recently, Fussell et al. introduced a new model for continuous learning with VR systems, based on the technology acceptance model (TAM) [7], which is linked to overall skill enhancement [10].

According to this model, "Attitude toward use" directly influences the trainee's commitment to training and skill development. This attitude is connected to "perceived usefulness" and "perceived ease of use" of the training system. "Perceived usefulness" refers to the extent to which a user believes that using VR for training will enhance their performance. "Perceived ease of use" is defined as the degree to which a user believes that using VR for training will require minimal effort. This encompasses not only the system's usability and ease of operation but also the mental effort required to use it.

In line with this model, we identified new factors related to real-time feedback that impact both perceived usefulness and perceived ease of use. "Perceived usefulness" is anticipated to be linked with "perceived behavior change," which measures the extent to which users believe that feedback has improved their subsequent behavior. This reflects a subjective, short-term effect of the training. To maintain "perceived ease of use," feedback should not disrupt the presentation process. This is termed the "disturbance level for feedback," which indicates "the extent to which feedback interferes with the ongoing presentation activity." The timing of feedback can influence these two subjective factors. Figure 6 presents a preliminary model summarizing these relationships.

3.2.3 Observable Information

The experiment below confirms the possibility of estimation of subjective values described in Sect. 3.2 from observable information. Although many studies have examined the predictability of performance and anxiety levels during presentations (e.g., [35–37]), there is no other study that has evaluated the impression for each of real-time feedback separately. Therefore, in this study, multimodal information such as voice, body movement, gaze, and physiological data were collected in an exploratory manner, taking into account the information used in the above studies.

3.3 *Experimental System*

3.3.1 Overview of the System

The system utilized was an adaptation of the experimental setup described in Sect. 2. Figure 7 illustrates the view of the virtual environment from the user's perspective. While various methods have been explored to automatically identify areas for improvement in presentations based on observed data, the accuracy of the current system often falls short compared to human judgment. Given this limitation, we chose to implement a Wizard of Oz (WoZ) approach, where a human evaluator identifies and points out areas that require improvement. Specifically, the system was designed so that the evaluator can provide feedback to the trainee via keyboard input whenever an improvement point is observed. Upon pressing a key, the trainee receives a corresponding icon indicating the feedback, with a delay ranging from 0 to 5 seconds, uniformly distributed to gather diverse timing data. After completing their presentation, trainees rated each piece of feedback they received. During the experiment, various data, including body movements, eye gaze, voice, heart rate, perspiration, and slide transitions, were continuously recorded. Additionally, the E4 wristband was used to measure perspiration and heart rate, capturing data every second. This data was first stored on the device and then uploaded to a dedicated cloud service.

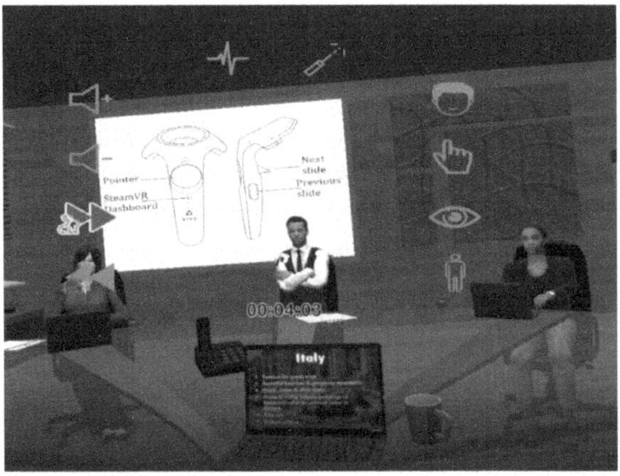

Fig. 7 User's view in the training environment

3.3.2 Feedback Method

In this study, to specifically focus on the timing of feedback, only one type of feedback method was used—a simple icon, similar to the approach by Palmas et al. [27]. According to the Presentation Evaluation Metrics provided by Human Global Communications Co., Ltd. 1, ten types of icons were defined. These icons can be broadly categorized into three groups: (1) Voice, which includes indicators for increasing or decreasing loudness based on voice volume and speech speed, respectively; (2) Physical Behavior, which encompasses elements such as smiling, eye contact, hand movements, and body posture; and (3) Presentation Skills, which relates to the appropriateness of speech inflection and pointer use.

Real-time feedback can become counterproductive if it frequently and excessively disrupts the ongoing training. However, feedback must also be sufficiently noticeable to the user. The intensity of icon presentation was adjusted based on parameters including size, position, duration, and the method of stimulus change during the presentation.

Through iterative preliminary experiments and adjustments conducted by three graduate students, the final parameters were determined. As depicted in Fig. 7, the ten icons were always displayed in gray within the HMD coordinate system, positioned to avoid the central field of view (as seen in [19]). Each icon flashed red twice and then stayed red for five seconds to signal to the user that a related issue had been identified. After this period, the icon color returned to gray, and the next keystroke was accepted. To prevent confusion, no more than two icons were shown simultaneously.

3.3.3 Recorded Data

Six types of information were recorded during the experiment in the following format:

(1) Audio was recorded as a common wav file.
(2) Body posture and movements were recorded by Microsoft's Azure Kinect at 30 fps as the 3D position and rotation in the Kinect depth camera coordinate system for 25 joints, excluding joints on the face.[2]
(3) Eye gaze was determined by the vector created from the approximate intersection of the gaze directions of the right and left eyes, combined with the midpoint. between the right and left eyes, as provided by the eye camera SDK in the Vive Pro Eye. This gaze information was recorded at a rate of 60 frames per second.
(4) Blood Volume Pulse (BVP) was recorded at 64 fps by the E4 wristband. In addition, Electrodermal Activity (EDA) was recorded at 4 fps by the same device.
(5) Slide switching is performed by the key operation of the VR controller in the user's hand. All keystroke timings and page numbers were recorded.
(6) The user completed a pre-experiment questionnaire rating their anxiety and public speaking skills on three levels.

---

[2] https://human-gc.jp/english/

Additionally, the times when the evaluator pressed the key to present the feedback icon when the icon was actually displayed after the delay, and the type of icon were all recorded.

3.4 Experiment

3.4.1 Overview

Participants wore the HMD and gave presentations in a virtual space. The evaluator (experimenter) always observed the presentation, and if she found behavior to be improved, she made keystrokes corresponding to each feedback icon (Fig. 7: Experimenter's viewpoint during the experiment). Icons were presented in front of the participants' view, and based on these, they were asked to improve their behavior without stopping their presentations. Immediately following their presentations, participants were shown a video recording of their views in the virtual environment and asked to respond to their scores for each piece of feedback received. After the experiment, the impact of the feedback was qualitatively confirmed by observing the presenter's behavior and voice immediately after the real-time feedback in the recorded video. In addition, the relationship between each subjective score and the observable information was analyzed to ascertain if it is possible to estimate undesirable timing for participants.

3.4.2 Participants

Eighteen participants (all graduate students in information science and materials science, all non-native English speakers, 8 males and 10 females, aged 27–37 years ($M = 28.61$, $SD = 4.30$) at a local university were recruited by email to participate in this study. While none were native English speakers, all participants had an English proficiency level above pre-advanced, indicating they could speak and understand well but still made mistakes and were sometimes not clearly understood. According to a pre-presentation questionnaire, four participants reported low anxiety levels when giving presentations, six reported medium anxiety, and eight reported high anxiety. Each participant received an honorarium of 2,000 JPY for their two hours of work in the experiment.

3.4.3 Procedures

First, the experimenter provided an overview of the experiment and obtained informed consent from each participant. Baseline measurements of Blood Volume Pulse (BVP) and Electrodermal Activity (EDA) were recorded for 5 minutes. Participants were seated in a chair and equipped with a Head-Mounted Display (HMD) and an E4 wristband. To facilitate relaxation, a high-fidelity meditation platform called Meditation VR 2 on Steam was used. Following this, each participant received instructions on how to use the system and how to deliver their presentation using it. The eye tracker was then calibrated, and the experimenter ensured that each participant had sufficient time to familiarize themselves with the system. Participants were specifically asked to remember the meaning of each feedback icon.

After setting up the system, participants were asked to choose one slide from a selection of ten slides across five topics (food, lifestyle, spirituality, sports, travel). They were given 10 minutes to organize their presentations without wearing the HMD, followed by 5 minutes of free practice while wearing the HMD. After this initial training, the participants began their presentations and the system began recording the data when the experimenter signaled the start of the training session. The evaluator (experimenter) observed the situation and, following the presentation metric, made keystrokes corresponding to each piece of feedback once she found improvement points. Each presentation was five to seven minutes long.

Immediately after each presentation, participants responded to each feedback with subjective scores in Sect. 5.4 while watching their own viewpoint videos during the training. After a 10-minute break, the above procedure was repeated with another presentation topic. Finally, a brief interview was conducted to obtain opinions on the feedback method and the training effectiveness of the system.

3.4.4 Subjective Scores

The scores to which the participants responded for each feedback after each presentation are listed below (See Sect. 3.2.2). Each score was answered on a five-point scale.

(1) Perceived behavior changing (PBC): How much did you change your behavior according to the feedback you received? 1: Nothing changed. 3: I changed my behavior once but forgot about it soon. 5: I changed my behavior immediately, and kept it in mind for the whole presentation.
(2) Disturbance level for feedback (DL): How much did this feedback disturb or distract you? 1: Not disturbed/distracted at all. 3: It disturbed/distracted me little, but I can deal with it. 5: It disturbed/distracted me a lot, and even interrupted the presentation for a while.

Note that PBC is the effect of feedback until the end of the presentation, and DL is the impression of feedback immediately after receiving it.[3]

[3] https://store.steampowered.com/app/1301850/MeditationVR/

3.5 Results

The total number of feedbacks presented to all participants was 228. Excluding nine unnoticed feedbacks and four feedbacks with eye tracker errors, the remaining 215 feedbacks were analyzed.

3.5.1 Negative Impact of Feedback on Presentation

We qualitatively analyzed the observable disturbing effect of the feedback on the ongoing presentation. The experimenter checked observable changes in the presentation for 15 seconds after each of the feedback with the recorded audio and video. The following three main negative effects were observed (See Fig.8a). The first is the case that the presenter suddenly stops speaking for more than three seconds immediately after presenting feedback (even though it is not during the slide changeover, etc.). The sudden speech stop gives a rather negative impression to the audience when it occurs in a real presentation. Such cases were observed 35 times (/ 215). The second is the case of a clear increase in filler words (e.g., Uh, well). Due to individual differences in the frequency of filler word use, we considered a negative case to be one in which the use of filler words increased by more than twice in the 15 seconds immediately after the feedback, compared to the 15 seconds before the feedback. Such cases were observed 33 times (/ 215). The third was the repetition of the same word. We considered this case when the same two or more words were repeated within 15 seconds after the feedback. Such cases were observed 16 times. In some instances, these three cases occurred simultaneously, resulting in a total of 65 occurrences out of 215 where any negative effect was observed. In other words, in as many as 30% of the cases, a negative impact (observable by the audience) was noticed on the presenter immediately after the feedback.

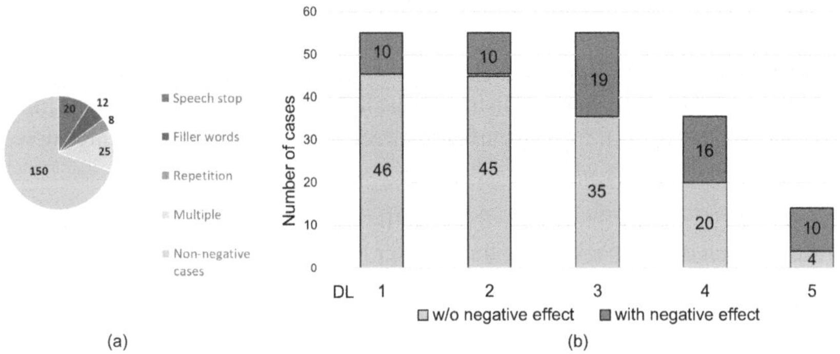

Fig. 8 Negative effects of real-time feedback. **a** Types of negative effects. **b** Number of cases with negative effects included in each disturbance level (DL)

The Pearson's correlation coefficient between its occurrence and the DL score was 0.36 ($p < 0.01$). There was no significant correlation between its occurrence and PBC.

3.5.2 Estimation of Perceived Behavior Change and Disturbance Level for Feedback

Simple models to estimate each score (i.e., PBC and DL) were created from all the recorded multimodal data with the Random Forest. A 10-fold cross-validation was performed using the 215 data. For PBC, the correlation coefficient was 0.45. The correlation coefficient for DL was 0.56. On the other hand, adding the participants' property data (i.e., anxiety level as described in Sect. 3.3.3) and the icon type improved the correlation coefficient to 0.53 for PBC, and 0.62 for DL.

3.5.3 Detection of Feedback Timing that Negatively Impacts Presenters

Finally, we describe the possibility of predicting feedback that could have a negative impact by using the DL values. Only DL was used for this estimation because PBC was not correlated with the occurrence of negatively affected feedback. Figure 8b shows the number of cases with negative effects included in each DL value. The higher the DL value, the higher the percentage of cases that had a negative impact at a given DL value. From this result, for example, if feedback is not displayed simply when the DL is greater than or equal to 3, 70 % (19 + 16 − 10 + 65) negative cases can be avoided. Similarly, by using the estimated DLs in Section 6.4, 62% negative cases (40 65) can be avoided. However, note that this is the result of fitting the model to the test data.

3.6 Limitations and Future Work

In this experiment, we showed that real-time feedback can negatively influence participants' behavior in the immediate aftermath and that some of this can be estimated from the multimodal information immediately prior to the feedback.

At present, however, this study presents several unexplored issues that leave gaps for future research. First, all participants in this study are graduate students, and the results are therefore specific to this demographic. It is essential to enrich the data by conducting the same experiment with participants of diverse backgrounds. Additionally, developing individual models for each participant represents a potential avenue for future research.

The features calculated using the measured data are rudimentary and need to be replaced with more sophisticated ones, such as those derived from combining multiple data sources. For example, the results indicated that the timing of looking at the slides was negatively associated with DL. However, if the speaker is speaking fluently, the timing of slide viewing might not lead to a lower DL. In such cases, this timing could potentially be detected by integrating head direction and voice information.

Additionally, it is crucial to verify whether withdrawing feedback at times that negatively affect presentations during training genuinely leads to improvements. Conversely, the reverse could also be true, as alternative training strategies, such as overload training, might be effective. We plan to conduct an experiment using a system that provides real-time feedback based on DL to assess its training effects as the next step.

4 Summary of Contributions in This Chapter

In this chapter, we explored the use of VR technology for reflection on one's own performance and real-time feedback as applied to public speaking.

Reflection on one's own performance in VR takes advantage of the characteristics of being able to change one's viewpoint on VR (from a first-person perspective) and of being able to change one's own appearance to a different appearance. As a result, VR reflection proved to be particularly effective for those who lacked confidence in public speaking.

Real-time feedback in VR takes advantage of the property that multimodal information about the user, observable in the VR environment, can be used for both problem-finding and internal estimation. As a result, it is clear that real-time feedback in VR should only be presented at appropriately selected times, as the timing of its presentation can have negative effects.

Although public speaking was used as a case study in this study, these studies were designed with care to ensure that they are easily generalizable. Therefore, it is expected that they will be transferable to other similar communication training (e.g., social skills training).

5 Competing Interests

The authors have no conflicts of interest to declare that are relevant to the content of this chapter.

6 Ethics Approval

The user study was conducted in accordance with the Helsinki Declaration guidelines. Ethical approval was obtained from the review board of Nara Institute of Science and Technology (Reference No.2019-I-29, No.2021-I-23), and we obtained informed consent from all participants.

References

1. E. Aronson, R.M. Akert, T. D. Wilson, *Social Psychology*. Pearson Prentice Hall., (2007)
2. L. Aymerich-Franch, J. Bailenson, The use of doppelgangers in virtual reality to treat public speaking anxiety: a gender comparison. In Proceedings of the International Society for Presence Research Annual Conference, (Citeseer 2014), pp. 173–186
3. L. Batrinca, G. Stratou, A. Shapiro, L.P. Morency, S. Scherer, *Cicero-towards a multimodal virtual audience platform for public speaking training*. In International Workshop on Intelligent Virtual Agents, (Springer 2013), pp. 116–128
4. J. Bourhis, M. Allen, The role of videotaped feedback in the instruction of public speaking: a quantitative synthesis of published empirical research. Commun. Res. Rep. **15**(3), 256–261 (1998)
5. M. Chollet, P. Ghate, C. Neubauer, S. Scherer, *Influence of individual differences when training public speaking with virtual audiences*. In Proceedings of the 18th International Conference on Intelligent Virtual Agents, pp. 1–7. (2018)
6. I. Damian, C.S.S. Tanz, T. Baur, J. Schoning, K. Luyten, E. Andre´, *Augustmenting social interactions: Realtime behavioural feedback using social signal processing techniques*. In Proceedings of International Conference on Human Factors in Computing Systems (2015), CHI '15, ACM, pp. 565–574
7. F.D. Davis, R.P. Bagozzi, P.R. Warshaw, User acceptance of computer technology: a comparison of two theoretical models. Manage. Sci. **35**(8), 982–1003 (1989)
8. Y. Fujimoto, Z. Hangyu, T. Sawabe, M. Kanbara, H. Kato, *Stop bad real-time feedback!: estimation of the timing of feedback that negatively impacts presenters for presentation training in virtual reality*. In Proceedings of The 22nd IEEE International Symposium on Mixed and Augmented Reality, ISMAR2023, IEEE, (2023)
9. T. Furmark, M. Tilfors, P.O. Everz, Social phobia in the general population: prevalence and sociodemographic profile. Soc. Psychiatr. Psychiatr. Epidemiol. **34**(8), 416–424 (1999)
10. S.G. Fussell, D. Truong, Using virtual reality for dynamic learning: an extended technology acceptance model. Virtual Reality **26**(1), 249–267 (2021)
11. A. Gaibani, F. Elmenfi, The role of gender in influencing public speaking anxiety. Br. J. Engl. Linguist. **2**(3), 7–13 (2014)
12. H. Gilkinson, Social fears reported by students in college speech classes. Speech Monogr. **9**(1), 131–160 (1942)
13. G. Gorisse, O. Christmann, E.A. Amato, S. Richir, First-and third-person perspectives in immersive virtual environments: presence and performance analysis of embodied users. Front. Robot. AI **4**, 33 (2017)
14. Z. Hangyu, Y. Fujimoto, M. Kanbara, H. Kato, *Effectiveness of virtual reality playback in public speaking training*. In Proceedings of Workshop on Social Affective Multi- modal Interaction for Health in 22nd ACM International Conference on Multimodal Interaction (ICMI2020), SAMIH '20, ACM, (2020)
15. J.N. Hook, C.A. Smith, D.P. Valentiner, A short-form of the personal report of confidence as a speaker. Pers. Individ. Differ. **44**(6), 1306–1313 (2008)

16. C.L. Hoyt, J. Blascovich, K.R. Swinth, Social inhibition in immersive virtual environments. Presence Teleoperators Virtual Environ. **12**(2), 183–195 (2003)
17. S.T. Iqbal, B.P. Bailey, *Investigating the effectiveness of mental workload as a predictor of opportune moments for interruption*. In Proceedings of the SIGCHI Conference on Human Factors in Computing Systems (CHI'05), pp. 1489–1492. (2005)
18. H. Iriye, P.L.S. Jacques, Memories for third-person experiences in immersive virtual reality. Sci. Rep. **11**(1), 1–14 (2021)
19. N. Janaka, C. Haigh, H. Kim, S. Zhang, S. Zhao, *Paracentral and near-peripheral visualizations: Towards attention- maintaining secondary information presentation on OHMDS during in-person social interactions*. In Proceedings of the SIGCHI Conference on Human Factors in Computing Systems (CHI'22), pp. 1–14. (2022)
20. I.L. Kampmann, P.M. Emmelkamp, D. Hartanto, W.P. Brinkman, B.J. Zijlstra, N. Morina, Exposure to virtual social interactions in the treatment of social anxiety disorder: a randomized controlled trial. Behav. Res. Ther. **77**, 147–156 (2016)
21. K.A. Karl, J.M. Kopf, Will individuals who need to improve their performance the most, volunteer to receive videotaped feedback? J. Bus. Commun. **31**(3), 213–223 (1973)
22. K. Kilteni, R. Groten, M. Slater, VR facial animation via multiview image translation. Presence Teleoperators Virtual Environ., 21, 4 (2012)
23. P.E. King, M.J. Young, R.R. Behnke, Public speaking performance improvement as a function of information processing in immediate and delayed feedback interventions. Commun. Educ. **49**, 365–374 (2000)
24. M.N. Levitan, E.M. Falcone, M. Placido, S. Krieger, L. Pinheiro, J.A. Crippa, L.M. Bruno, D. Pastore, J. Hallak, A.E. Nardi, Public speaking in social phobia: a pilot study of self-ratings and observers' ratings of social skills. J. Clin. Psychol. **68**(4), 397–402 (2012)
25. Ltd., V. Virtual speech, September (2017)
26. F. Mostajeran, M.B. Balci, F. Steinicke, S. Kuhn, J. Gallinat, *The effects of virtual audience size on social anxiety during public speaking*. In Proceedings of IEEE Conference on Virtual Reality and 3D User Interfaces, VR '20, IEEE, pp. 303–312. (2020)
27. F. Palmas, R. Reinelt, J.E. Cichor, D.A. Plecher, G. Klinker, *Virtual reality public speaking training: Experimental evaluation of direct feedback technology acceptance*. In Proceedings of the IEEE Virtual Reality and 3D User Interfaces, pp. 463–472. (2021)
28. J. Schneider, D. Börner, P. Van Rosmalen, M. Specht, Presentation trainer: what experts and computers can tell about your nonverbal communication. J. Comput. Assist. Learn. **33**(2), 164–177 (2017)
29. L.M. Schreiber, G.D. Paul, L.R. Shibley, The development and test of the public speaking competence rubric. Commun. Educ. **61**(3), 205–233 (2012)
30. S. Stupar-Rutenfrans, L.E. Ketelaars, M.S. van Gisbergen, Beat the fear of public speaking: Mobile 360 video virtual reality exposure training in home environment reduces public speaking anxiety. Cyberpsychol. Behav. Soc. Netw. **20**(10), 624–633 (2017)
31. Technologies, V. H. Virtual orator, (2015)
32. V. Tejwani, D. Ha, C. Isada, Observations: public speaking anxiety in graduate medical education-a matter of interpersonal and communication skills? J. Grad. Med. Educ. **8**(1), 111 (2016)
33. S. Torres-Guijarro, M. Bengoechea, Gender differential in self-assessment: a fact neglected in higher education peer and self-assessment techniques. High. Educ. Res. Dev. **36**(5), 1072–1084 (2017)
34. S. Walker, T. Weidner, K.J. Armstrong, Standardized patient encounters and individual case-based simulations improve students' confidence and promote reflection: a preliminary study. Athl. Train. Educ. J. **10**(2), 130–137 (2015)
35. T. Wo¨rtwein, M. Chollet, B. Schauerte, L.P. Morency, R. Stiefelhagen, S. Scherer, *Multimodal public speaking performance assessment*. In Proceedings of ACM on International Conference on Multimodal Interaction (ICMI '15), pp. 43–50. (2015)
36. T. Wo¨rtwein, L.P. Morency, S. Scherer, *Automatic assessment and analysis of public speaking anxiety: A virtual audience case study*. In Proceedings of International Conference on Affective Computing and Intelligent Interaction (ACII2015), pp. 187–193. (2015)

37. M. Yadav, M.N. Sakib, E.H. Nirjhar, K. Feng, A. Behzadan, T. Chaspari, Exploring individual differences of public speaking anxiety in real-life and virtual presentations. IEEE Trans. Affect. Comput., (2020)
38. H. Zhou, Y. Fujimoto, M. Kanbara, H. Kato, Virtual reality as a reflection technique for public speaking training. Appl. Sci. **11**, 9 (2021)

Introduces Interaction and Pedagogical Feedback

Interaction in Social Skills Training

Hiroki Tanaka and Satoshi Nakamura

Abstract Social communication is a crucial factor influencing human social life. Quantifying the degree of difficulty an individual faces in social communication is necessary to understand developmental and neurological disorders and to create systems for automatic screening as well as assistive methods such as social skills training (SST). As discussed elsewhere in this book, SST by experienced human trainers is a well-established method. In this chapter, we describe interaction in social skills training. Specifically, we present an analysis of the human social skills training dataset, the development of virtual SST, and the acceptability of this approach.

1 Introduction

Social skills training (SST) is frequently employed in psychiatric rehabilitation programs to enhance social skills. It is particularly effective for individuals who experience social challenges due to mental illnesses or developmental difficulties. Previous studies have identified several communication traits associated with schizophrenia and autism spectrum disorder (ASD). However, limited research has been conducted in natural conversational environments using computational features, since automatic capture and analysis in such settings are challenging. Despite these challenges, natural data collection holds significant potential for accurately identifying the true communication characteristics of individuals with mental difficulties and the differences between participants and trainers in their interactions. Consequently, we gathered a one-on-one SST multimodal dataset to explore and automatically capture the natural characteristics exhibited by individuals with mental conditions like schizophrenia or ASD as well as controls (typical development). To validate the dataset's potential, we used partially annotated data to train a classifier

H. Tanaka (✉)
International Christian University, Mitaka, Japan
e-mail: hiroki.tanaka@icu.ac.jp

S. Nakamura
Nara Institute of Science and Technology, Ikoma, Japan
e-mail: s-nakamura@is.naist.jp

S. Nakamura (ed.), *Multimodal Interaction Technologies for Training Affective Social Skills*, https://doi.org/10.1007/978-981-96-1313-7_10

for distinguishing between schizophrenia and controls using audiovisual features. This classification task, based solely on natural interaction data rather than data from specific clinical assessment tasks, achieved over 85% accuracy, precision, recall, and F1-score [1]. Furthermore, we introduce an analysis of the human social skills training dataset used, describe the development of automated SST, and discuss the acceptability of this approach.

2 SST Dataset

In this section, we present an analysis of the human social skills training dataset.

All data collection processes were approved by the ethical committees at Nara Medical University and Nara Institute of Science and Technology. At the beginning of recording sessions, we explained the procedure to the participants and obtained informed consent. To capture subtle social signals of the participants and trainers, we used three video cameras and two Azure Kinects. We installed transparent partitions between participants and trainers to prevent infections. Two cameras were placed diagonally to avoid light reflection from the partitions as they captured facial expressions, while the third camera was positioned centrally to capture the entire scene. The Kinects captured body movements with a pre-trained pose estimator based on depth images. The same workflow and devices were used throughout the data collection process.

To investigate interaction differences among individuals with various mental or developmental difficulties, we recruited participants with ASD, SZ, and controls (without ASD and SZ). While equalizing the environments across all recordings is ideal, our recordings were conducted at two different locations (university or hospital) to minimize the participants' mental anxiety. However, we made conscientious efforts to standardize other environmental factors. We focused on the four fundamental social skills defined by Bellack [2]: listening, speaking, declining a request, and making a request.

We collected data from 52 adult participants: 21 controls, 15 with ASD, and 16 with SZ. Additionally, we gathered data from 33 children (17 controls and 16 ASD) to more fully investigate ASD [3]. This chapter primarily describes the adult participants. All videos were synchronized by a human annotator using a handclap signal at the beginning and end of each role-play, and all utterances were transcribed by the annotator. Furthermore, we conducted an additional recording to analyze eye-gaze differences with the same participants on the same day for another research study [4]. All participants were native Japanese speakers, so the target language was Japanese.

3 Classification Analysis

We used the dataset to train a classifier that can handle multimodal features. For this empirical study, we focused on classifying adult control participants and adult SZ participants.

The random forest algorithm was adopted as our machine learning model. For its input, we employed audiovisual features calculated by conventional software and preprocessed the data with the following procedure. First, audio data were extracted from the video data. We then segmented the data according to SST phases, such as role-plays or feedback sessions. For the audio data, we removed unvoiced segments and segments with overlapping voices between the trainer and the participant, and then, we concatenated the non-overlapping voiced segments. Audio files shorter than five seconds were eliminated due to their inadequacy for accurate calculation. Note that body joint positions were not used because we have not yet synchronized this data at the boundary points of SST phases.

We used Praat for calculating audio features and OpenFace for calculating visual features. Tables 1 and 2 show the input features, where F0 represents the fundamental frequency of voiced segments, F1–F3 represent the first to third formants of voiced segments, and AUXX represents facial action units (AUs), which are components of facial expressions. Due to differing background noise levels at the various recording locations, we excluded the average, minimum, and maximum values of intensity to avoid location-based discrepancies, although we included the range and standard deviation, since they were possibly less affected.

All features were standardized to have a mean of zero and a standard deviation of one before being input to the model. To determine which modality was dominant for this classification, we used three different feature set conditions: audio-only (A), visual-only (V), and audiovisual (A + V). We trained the model ten times with random parameters and then averaged the results to obtain a final result.

Table 3 shows the classification results, with the highest F1-score being 0.887. Regarding modality differences, the audio-only features exhibited the best performance across all metrics, while the visual-only features performed significantly

Table 1 Audio features

Feature name	Description
F0, F1, F2, F3 mean	Mean frequency of F0, F1, F2, F3
F0, F1, F2, F3 SD	Standard deviation of F0, F1, F2, F3
F0 Min, Max	Minimum and maximum F0 frequency
F0 range	Range (Max–Min) of F0
F1, F2, F3 BW	Average bandwidth of F1, F2, F3
F2/F1, F3/F1 Mean	The mean ratio of F2-F1 and F3-F1
F2/F1, F3/F1 SD	Standard deviation of F2/F1 and F3/F1
Int range	Range (Max–Min) of intensities
Int SD	The standard deviation of vocal intensity

Table 2 Visual features

Feature name	Description
Pose_[R_x,R_y,R_z]_std	The standard deviation of head rotation around (*X*: pitch, *Y*: yaw, *Z*: roll) axis
Smile_ratio	Ratio of smiling frames
AU01	Inner-brow raiser
AU02	Outer-brow raiser
AU04	Brow lower
AU05	Upper-lid raiser
AU06	Cheek raiser
AU07	Lid tightener
AU09	Nose wrinkler
AU10	Upper-lip raiser
AU12	Lip-corner puller
AU15	Lip-corner depressor
AU17	Chin raiser
AU20	Lip stretcher
AU23	Lip tightener
AU25	Lips parted
AU26	Jaw dropper
AU28	Lip sucker
AU45	Blinker

worse. The audiovisual features demonstrated average performance. These results highlight the importance of audio features in distinguishing between the two groups. Additionally, we analyzed the importance of features using random forest and found that F3 BW had the highest importance value, more than double that of the other features. These datasets and models were further applied to automated social skills trainer + (Sect. 4.2) and the extended prediction models mentioned in Chapt. 7.

Table 3 Classification results [1]

Feature	Accuracy	Precision	Recall	F1-score	Feature set
A	0.868	0.902	0.872	**0.887**	A
V	0.382	0.476	0.488	0.422	V
A + V	0.804	0.823	0.851	0.836	A + V

4 Development of Virtual Agents: Social Skills Trainer

Previous studies have employed computers to train social skills, particularly in areas such as public speaking and emotion regulation. Another related line of research has focused on automated conversational coaches. For example, Hoque et al. [5] developed a dialogue system designed to help individuals enhance their interview skills by providing real-time feature detection and feedback. That system achieved several notable outcomes: (1) it set a realistic task for actual users, (2) it delivered formative and effective feedback with specific comments on behaviors needing improvement, and (3) it interpreted user utterances to inform the selection of backchannels or formative feedback.

Our proposed system adheres to the medically proven framework of SST, which includes (1) instruction and target skills, (2) modeling, (3) role-playing, (4) feedback, and (5) homework. We developed an automated social skills trainer that fully conforms to SST's basic training model through use of an embodied conversational agent [6].

4.1 *Multimodal System Implementation*

Social skills training is a long-established method that was originally developed to reduce anxiety and discomfort and obtain appropriate skills during social interaction [2].

SST can be classified into individual (one-to-one training) or group (one-to-many or many-to-many training) settings. One advantage of group SST is that it enables participants to observe the behaviors of other participants and receive feedback from others. On the other hand, the advantage of individual SST is that the training can be relaxed and simplified, and lessons can be tailored to individual needs.

The basic SST training model generally follows these steps: instruction, modeling, role-playing, feedback, and homework. We describe these steps and our system implementation.

The automated social skills trainer was developed from MMDAgent, a Japanese spoken dialogue system that integrates speech recognition, dialogue management, text-to-speech, and behavior generation. MMDAgent works as a Windows application.

1. **Instruction:** Instruction includes defining target skills and explaining their goals. After identifying the major social problems faced by the trainee, the skills to be learned are determined based on these problems. As an example of a target skill, the automatic social skills trainer sets a speaking task, which emphasizes telling positive stories, because narrating stories is important for other higher-level skills.
2. **Modeling:** Trainers act as models and demonstrate the skill on which the users are focusing so that they can see what they need to do before attempting it themselves. The automated social skills trainer replicates this step for speaking

skills by allowing users to watch a recorded video model of people with relatively good speaking skills. Users can watch and imitate such good examples.

3. **Role-playing:** Participants role-play a scene of the lesson's skill for the trainer. This allows them to practice their skills in the target situation. Trainers observe the participants' social skills and focus on voice quality, amplitude, facial expressions, eye gaze, and other non-verbal behaviors. In the automated social skills trainer, the users also perform role-plays. After the user says, "Start the role-play," the system says, "Please describe something fun you did recently." The role-playing starts after the system's request and continues for one minute. During this time, the agent nods its head, and the system automatically senses and analyzes the audiovisual features from the user's video (Fig. 1).
4. **Feedback:** Trainers provide feedback to help the participants identify their strengths and weaknesses. At the end of the role-playing, the automated social skills trainer immediately analyzes the features of the user's video and determines its feedback, which it then displays. Since displaying too many features in the feedback may confuse users, the system performs feature selection to identify effective features for defining speaking skills [7]. Based on the calculated features, the system displays feedback for the users. The following types of feedback are displayed in a simple way for greater comprehension and interpretation:

User video: Users can watch the recorded video and audio of their speech.

Overall score: The system displays a predicted overall score, which motivates users to practice and raise their scores. We predict the overall scores using the generalized linear multiple regression method on a scale from 0 to 100. Regarding the regression model's features, because our analysis of the data found that the smiling ratio of the video model was the highest, we added this ratio to the

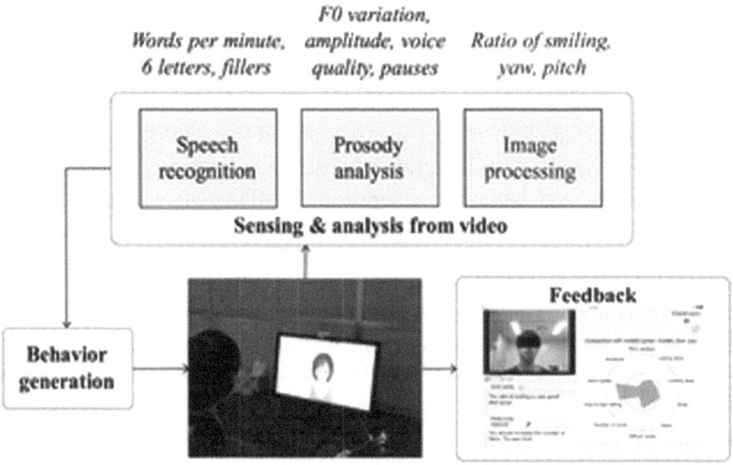

Fig. 1 System framework [6]

regression model's input features. We confirmed that the correlation coefficient between the predicted speaking skills and the subjectively evaluated skills using leave-one-user-out cross-validation was 0.55, which indicates a weak correlation when using statistically significant features: words per minute, amplitude, words over six letters, and smiling ratio.

Comparison with models: The system uses a radar chart to compare the extracted features between the user's current speech and the model persons' speeches in terms of z-score, a statistical measurement of a score's relationship to the mean within a group of scores.

Comments: The system generates positive comments that reinforce the user's motivation based on features whose values are the closest to those of the model. It also generates comments about points that need improvement based on a feature with a median distance from the model. This choice of median (instead of farthest) distance for the feature was based on discussions with a professional social skills trainer who noted that it might be fundamentally infeasible to expect people with social communication difficulties to improve their worst points [2].

Homework: Trainers assign relatively easy homework challenges that participants must complete on their own time throughout the week to facilitate the generalization of learned skills to daily life. The automated social skills trainer sets minor homework challenges that users must finish over the week. For example, the system instructs users to tell a story to others throughout the week and then informs them that they will be asked to talk about that experience in the next session.

4.2 Social Skills Trainer +

We updated the system using embodied conversational agents (Greta virtual agents) [8] and implemented a Japanese spoken dialogue system that integrates several components: Google speech recognition, dialogue management, CereProc TTS (featuring a Japanese female voice as a character named Yuki)/Google TTS, and behavior generation, including head nodding. The modules are connected through ActiveMQ, and the system operates in real time as a Windows application.

One advantage of our system is that it allows people to practice repeatedly at their own pace, unlike training with a human. The automated social skills trainer + include the following elements: (1) self-introduction, (2) instruction and motivation, (3) modeling, (4) role-playing, (5) feedback, and (6) homework and closing [9]. Detailed scenarios were developed by three psychiatrists with SST experience. The modeling component involved watching recorded videos of two types: three videos of bad modeling and five videos of good modeling. We selected a target training task for each role-play from the following four tasks: listening to others, conveying positive feelings, requesting from others, and declining a request.

The system records users' voices and images using a pin microphone and a webcam to sense user behavior. During role-plays, it perceives the user's utterances via speech recognition and responds based on keywords (yes/I understand/I have, etc.) prepared by rule-based dialogue scenarios. Services of Google Cloud Platform were used for the speech recognition and speech synthesis modules. If the keywords were not directly included in the speech recognition output, we used the Japanese version of the Bidirectional Encoder Representations from Transformers (BERT) model to calculate the cosine distances between corresponding embeddings and the target keywords at the sentence level, selecting the closest match. We continuously improved our response selection module through validation to minimize dialogue selection errors and timing failures.

After role-plays, the system extracted multimodal features using the Praat toolkit for speech processing, OpenFace and OpenPose for image processing, and Google speech recognition for textual feature recognition. We developed a score evaluator using role-playing videos that automatically predicts seven items: eye contact, body orientation, facial expression, voice modulation, clarity, fluency, and social appropriateness. These items were rated on a 5-point scale by psychiatrists based on user behavioral indicators, using multimodal features (Praat, OpenFace, and OpenPose) and BERT similarity scores between utterances spoken by the virtual agent and users. Random forests were employed to predict these features, with ground truth ratings provided by two psychiatrists. Our detailed prediction performance was previously reported, showing correlation coefficients between the ground truth and predicted values ranging from approximately 0.1–0.6 [3].

Based on the evaluation results, a radar chart, positive comments, and corrective comments were presented on a screen along with video clips, where the comments were read aloud by the virtual agent. The radar chart displays the evaluation values, with past training history represented by a different color. Positive reinforcement, such as verbal praise or rewards, is provided immediately after role-play rehearsals to highlight specific successful behaviors (Fig. 2). Even for the poorest performances, a genuinely positive aspect must be identified. The virtual agent and feedback are shown on digital signage (Fig. 3), with the feedback displayed on full screen after the calculations are complete.

5 Acceptability as Social Skills Trainers

Our research, along with studies conducted by other groups, has been focused on automating social skills training using virtual agents. This effort has resulted in the development of automated social skills training systems that closely resemble human-led social skills training by design. Our system incorporates video modeling of human behavior, real-time behavior recognition, and feedback, distinguishing it from other systems among the various types of conversational agents.

We previously validated the effectiveness of this training in both children and adults with ASD, as well as in the general population [6]. The automated social

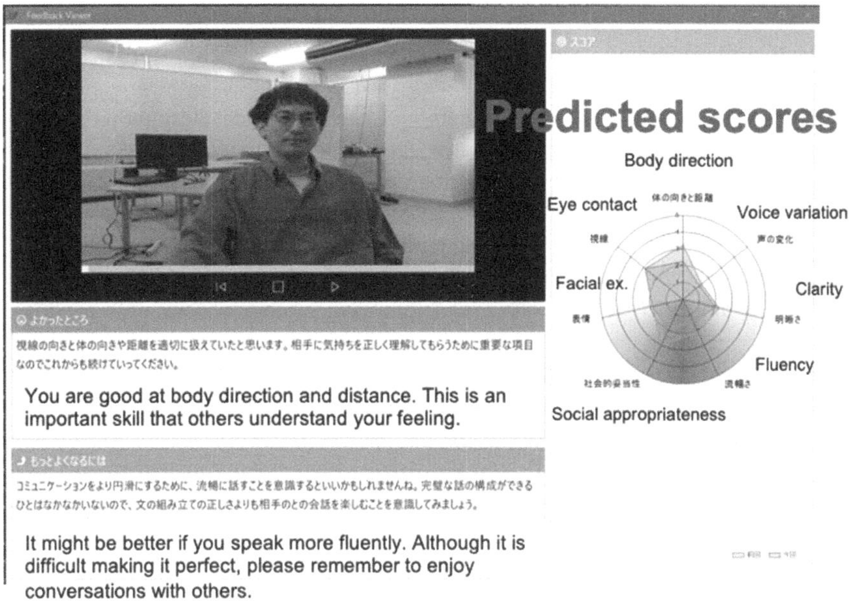

Fig. 2 Feedback window (translated into English)

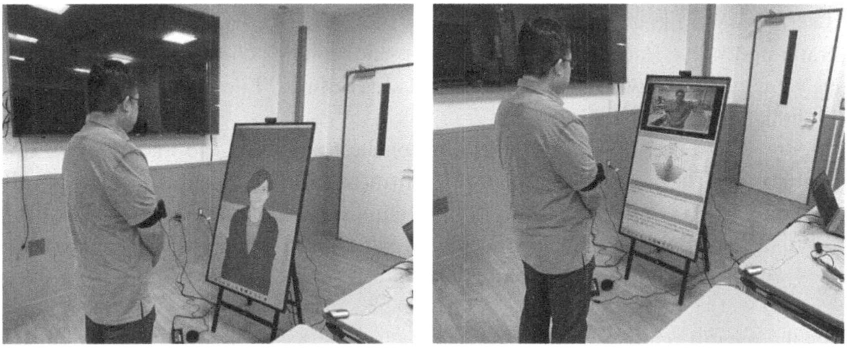

Fig. 3 Social skills training system (left: role-playing; right: feedback) [10]

skills training agent serves dual roles as a speaker and a listener. We found that this system was more effective in training social skills than traditional methods like reading books or watching videos of role models. Moreover, interacting with a virtual agent made users feel more comfortable and less tense compared to talking to a human [11].

However, the visual design of virtual agents, specifically which designs are more favored or accepted, has not been thoroughly investigated. Previous research has shown that the quality of the therapeutic alliance (i.e., the level of rapport and trust) is a reliable predictor of positive clinical outcomes, independent of the psychotherapy approach used (including social skills training and cognitive behavioral therapy) or the specific outcome measure [12].

We focus on comparing virtual agents with varying visual designs rather than comparing humans and robots in assistive technology, since virtual agent designs are easier to create and modify. The visual design of virtual agents in social skills training has been explored in previous research, although not comprehensively. For instance, Hoque et al. [5] matched male participants with male coaches and female participants with female coaches to reduce gender-based behavioral variability. In contrast, Tanaka et al. [6] didnotconsider the agent's gender, using only a female design.

Our study applies these findings and rating measures to investigate the design of our virtual agents, aiming to develop a more favorable and acceptable design for automated social skills training. To the best of our knowledge, no previous work has examined the visual design of virtual agents for automated social skills training, including the relationships between acceptability and other measures or those between likeability and individual user characteristics.

For data collection, we recruited participants from a crowdsourcing service (Crowdworks) [13]. The recruitment notice asked for participants 18 years of age or older with Japanese nationality. Data were collected to investigate the realism of the videos, as well as autistic traits. The questionnaire items measured the acceptability of the agent as a trainer and as a listener; its realism, familiarity, trustworthiness, and eeriness; the likeability of its face, eyes, hair, perceived age, and voice; and its overall impression. Each question was answered through a Google Form. The questions were evaluated with a 5-point Likert scale (from 1, "I don't think so at all," to 5, "I think so very much").

Figure 4 also presents the acceptability of the trainer and the likeability of the virtual agents. The Kruskal–Wallis test confirmed significant differences across all measures ($P < 0.001$). While there was a slight difference in the evaluation of likeability between the high and low social responsiveness scale (SRS) score groups (Fig. 4, lower right), the Wilcoxon rank-sum test revealed no significant difference (agent 1, $P = 0.13$; agent 6, $P = 0.25$) and indicated a small effect size. Figure 5 illustrates the overall realism ratings for the agents. The Kruskal–Wallis test indicated significant differences in the perceived realism of the virtual agents ($P < 0.001$), supporting our design assumption that agents 1 through 6 would be perceived as exhibiting progressively greater realism. These findings have been applied to the development of social skills trainers [10].

This chapter presented interaction in social skills training. We introduced an analysis of the human social skills training dataset, the development of automated social skills training, and the acceptability of this approach.

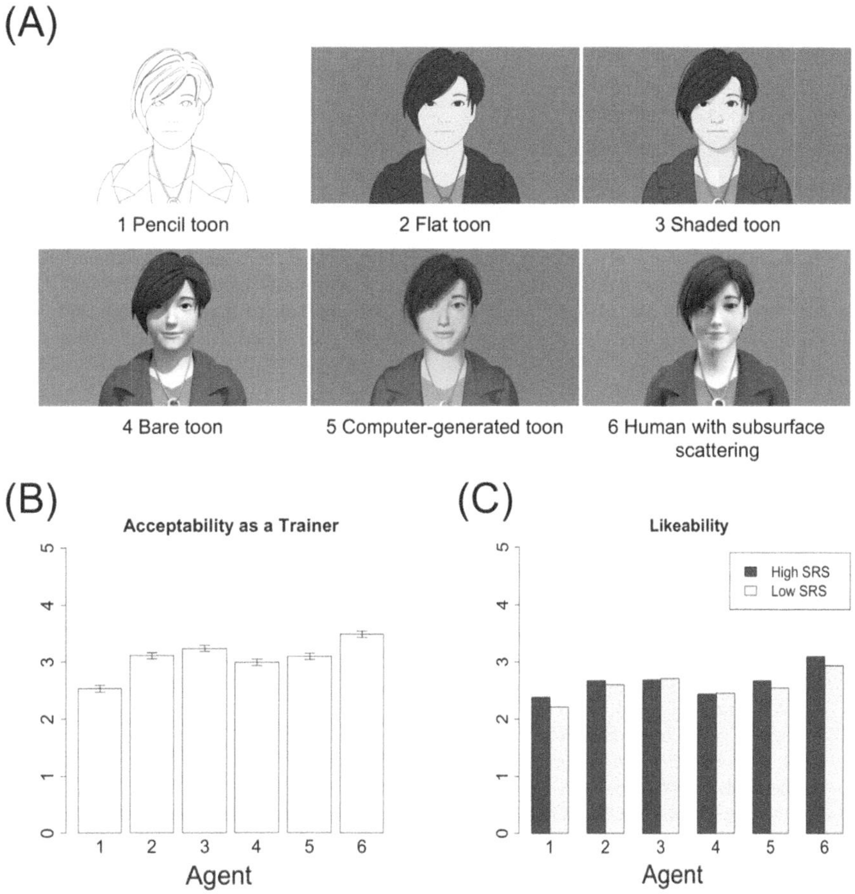

Fig. 4 Screen captures of the six virtual agents **a**; acceptability as a trainer (error bars represent standard error) **b**; and likeability evaluated by groups scored as having high and low autistic traits, measured by social responsiveness scale (SRS) **c** [2]

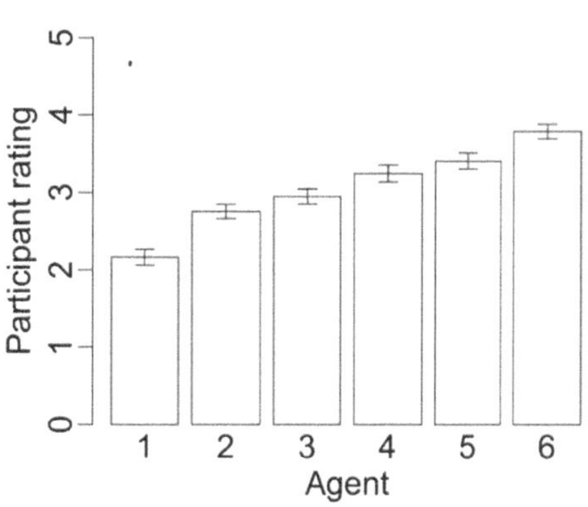

Fig. 5 Realism ratings. Error bars represent standard error [13]

Acknowledgements Most of the work done in this chapter was conducted at the Nara Institute of Science and Technology, Japan.

References

1. T. Saga, H. Tanaka, H. Iwasaka, Y. Matsuda, T. Morimoto, M. Uratani, S. Nakamura, *Multimodal dataset of social skills training in natural conversational setting*. In Companion Publication of the 2021 International Conference on Multimodal Interaction, (2021), pp. 395–399
2. K.T. Mueser, A.S. Bellack, S. Gingerich, J. Agresta, D. Fulford, Social skills training for schizophrenia. Guilford Publications. (2024)
3. T. Saga, H. Tanaka, Y. Matsuda, T. Morimoto, M. Uratani, K. Okazaki, S. Nakamura, Automatic evaluation-feedback system for automated social skills training. Sci. Rep. **13**(1), 6856 (2023)
4. K. Iwauchi, H. Tanaka, K. Okazaki, Y. Matsuda, M. Uratani, T. Morimoto, S. Nakamura, Eye-movement analysis on facial expression for identifying children and adults with neurodevelopmental disorders. Front. Digit. Health **5**, 952433 (2023)
5. M. Hoque, M. Courgeon, J.C. Martin, B. Mutlu, R.W. Picard, *Mach: My automated conversation coach*. In Proceedings of the 2013 ACM International Joint Conference on Pervasive and Ubiquitous Computing, pp. 697–706, (2013)
6. H. Tanaka, H. Negoro, H. Iwasaka, S. Nakamura, Embodied conversational agents for multimodal automated social skills training in people with autism spectrum disorders. PLoS ONE **12**(8), e0182151 (2017)
7. H. Zhou, Y. Fujimoto, M. Kanbara, H. Kato, Virtual reality as a reflection technique for public speaking training. Appl. Sci. **11**(9), 3988 (2021)
8. I. Poggi, C. Pelachaud, F. de Rosis, V. Carofiglio, B. De Carolis, Greta. *A believable embodied conversational agent*. In Multimodal Intelligent Information Presentation. Dordrecht: Springer Netherlands. (2005), pp. 3–25
9. H. Tanaka, H. Iwasaka, Y. Matsuda, K. Okazaki, S. Nakamura, Analyzing self-efficacy and summary feedback in automated social skills training. IEEE Open J. Eng. Med. Biol. **2**, 65–70 (2021)
10. H. Tanaka, T. Saga, K. Iwauchi, M. Honda, T. Morimoto, Y. Matsuda, S. Nakamura, The validation of automated social skills training in members of the general population over 4 weeks: Comparative study. JMIR Formative Res. **7**(1), e44857 (2023)
11. H. Tanaka, S. Sakriani, G. Neubig, T. Toda, H. Negoro, H. Iwasaka, S. Nakamura (2016) Teaching social communication skills through human-agent interaction. ACM Trans. Interact. Intell. Syst. **6**(2), 1–26. https://doi.org/10.1145/2937757
12. R.B. Ardito, D. Rabellino, Therapeutic alliance and outcome of psychotherapy: historical excursus, measurements, and prospects for research. Front. Psychol. **2**, 270 (2011)
13. H. Tanaka, S. Nakamura, The acceptability of virtual characters as social skills trainers: usability study. JMIR Hum. Factors **9**(1), e35358 (2022)

Interaction in Cognitive Behavioral Therapy

Kazuhiro Shidara and Takashi Kudo

Abstract Cognitive Behavioral Therapy (CBT) is a widely recognized and practical approach for treating various mental health issues, including depression, anxiety, and stress-related disorders. By focusing on identifying and restructuring negative thought patterns and behaviors, CBT empowers individuals to develop healthier coping mechanisms. Traditionally administered through face-to-face sessions with trained therapists, CBT has proven efficacy but faces barriers that limit its accessibility, such as limited availability of professionals, high costs, and geographical constraints. In this chapter, we address these limitations by presenting an adaptive Embodied Conversational Agent (ECA) that adjusts its questioning strategy based on the user's real-time psychological distress. By integrating a distress detection model analyzing users' speech transcriptions, the ECA personalizes the therapeutic interaction to ensure that interventions are neither overwhelming nor insufficient. We conducted an experiment with 49 participants, comparing an adaptive condition—where the number of Socratic questions was modified according to detected distress—with a random condition. Results demonstrated that the adaptive approach yielded superior outcomes in reducing psychological distress and negative moods. These findings highlight the potential of ECAs to offer CBT sessions for a broader population.

K. Shidara (✉)
Fujitsu Limited, Kawasaki, Japan
e-mail: s-kazuhiro@fujitsu.com

T. Kudo
Osaka University, Suita, Japan

S. Nakamura (ed.), *Multimodal Interaction Technologies for Training Affective Social Skills*, https://doi.org/10.1007/978-981-96-1313-7_11

1 Introduction

1.1 Conversational Agents for Cognitive Behavior Therapy

Cognitive Behavioral Therapy (CBT) is a widely recognized and practical approach for treating various mental health issues, including depression, anxiety, and stress-related disorders [1, 2]. By focusing on identifying and restructuring negative thought patterns and behaviors, CBT empowers individuals to develop healthier coping methods [3]. Traditionally administered through face-to-face sessions with trained therapists, CBT has proven efficacy but faces barriers that limit its accessibility [4]. Factors such as limited availability of trained professionals, high costs, geographical constraints, and psychological stigma often prevent individuals from seeking or receiving adequate mental health care.

The rise of technology, especially in artificial intelligence and conversation agents, has created new opportunities for providing CBT [5–7]. Embodied Conversational Agents (ECAs) are capable of human-like interactions with users through natural language processing (NLP), speech recognition, and responsive behaviors [8]. These agents offer a promising solution to bridge gaps in mental health care accessibility by providing scalable, affordable, and anonymous therapeutic interventions. By leveraging ECAs, it becomes possible to reach a broader population that might benefit from CBT but is underserved by traditional methods.

1.2 Challenges in Interaction Adapted to the User's State

While ECAs have shown promise in delivering CBT techniques, there remains a significant gap in how these ECAs adapt to individual users' psychological states during therapy sessions. In traditional CBT, therapists dynamically adjust their interventions based on real-time assessments of the client's distress levels, mood, and engagement. Existing ECAs might need more adaptability, potentially limiting their effectiveness.

Previous studies have implemented key therapeutic techniques such as Socratic questioning [9] in human-agent interaction. For instance, Kimani et al. [10] developed an ECA that utilized Socratic questions to reduce anxiety related to public speaking, providing questions based on a hierarchical, rule-based dialogue engine that presents multiple-choice inputs according to the dialogue context. Additionally, our previous study [11] compared scenarios with and without Socratic questioning and found that users who engaged with the questioning experienced greater reductions in negative moods. These studies suggest that ECAs can effectively replicate key therapeutic techniques of CBT.

However, these approaches do not account for the dynamic adaptation of the therapeutic process based on the user's psychological state. Specifically, limited research exists on ECAs that select system utterances in response to real-time estimation of user's psychological states. Addressing this gap is essential for enhancing the personalization and effectiveness of ECAs in delivering CBT.

This chapter presents our research [12] on developing an adaptive ECA that adjusts its questioning strategy based on the user's psychological distress level. By integrating a psychological distress detection model [13], an ECA can estimate the user's distress in real time and modify the number of Socratic questions accordingly. This approach aims to personalize the therapeutic interaction, ensuring that interventions are neither overwhelming nor insufficient, enhancing cognitive change, and distress reduction.

2 The Role of Socratic Questioning in CBT with an ECA

Socratic questioning [9] is a foundational technique in CBT that facilitates cognitive restructuring by encouraging individuals to critically evaluate their automatic thoughts and beliefs [2]. Originating from the pedagogical methods of the ancient Greek philosopher Socrates, this approach involves a series of guided questions that help clients explore the evidence behind their thoughts, consider alternative perspectives, and develop more balanced cognitions. By challenging cognitive distortions, Socratic questioning enables clients to gain insights into their thought patterns, leading to emotional relief and behavioral change.

In the context of ECAs, Socratic questioning can be systematized to provide consistent and structured therapeutic interventions. ECAs can employ predefined templates and adaptive algorithms to pose relevant questions that guide users through the cognitive restructuring process. This method not only promotes self-reflection but also empowers users to become active participants in their mental health care. By simulating the interactive dialogue of a human therapist, ECAs can effectively engage users in therapeutic conversations.

3 Adapting Response Selection to User's Psychological States

Effective therapeutic interactions require personalization and responsiveness to the user's current emotional and cognitive states. In human-delivered CBT, therapists adjust their interventions based on observations of the client's mood, distress levels, and readiness to engage in cognitive restructuring. Translating this adaptability to ECAs involves equipping ECAs with the ability to detect and interpret users' psychological states dynamically.

One approach to achieving this adaptability is through psychological distress detection models that analyze transcriptions of user inputs to estimate their level of psychological distress. By integrating these models, ECAs can adapt their questioning strategies, adjusting the number and type of Socratic questions posed based on the user's real-time emotional state. This ensures that the intervention is neither overwhelming nor insufficient, enhancing the likelihood of cognitive change and distress reduction.

For example, if a user exhibits high levels of distress, the agent employs additional Socratic questions, gradually guiding the user. Conversely, if the user shows signs of lower distress, the agent proceeds more directly by prompting the user to think of alternative thoughts. This adaptive interaction mirrors the theory of the cognitive model and is crucial for effectiveness.

Implementing such adaptability requires robust detection mechanisms and a flexible dialogue system capable of modifying its behavior based on user feedback. Our research focuses on developing an ECA that incorporates a psychological distress detection model to adjust its questioning strategy in real time, addressing the gap in existing ECAs.

4 System Design for Response Selection

In our study, we focused on integrating psychological state detection models based on the Kessler Psychological Distress Scale (K6) [14] to adjust questioning strategies and improve cognitive and emotional outcomes for users.

4.1 Overview of the Adaptive CBT System

Our system employs an ECA capable of conducting a CBT session through spoken dialogue. The agent interacts with users by guiding them through the identification of automatic thoughts, correcting ones, and fostering the development of balanced alternative thoughts. The system architecture includes components for speech recognition, NLP, dialogue management, and real-time psychological state detection.

The ECA is implemented using the Greta platform. To enhance user acceptance, especially among Japanese users, the agent's appearance was customized based on culturally appropriate design principles. We employed Google's Text-to-Speech API to generate synthesized speech with a Japanese female voice, ensuring natural and engaging interactions.

The CBT process implemented in our system involves three main steps:

- **Identifying Automatic Thoughts**: The agent guides the user to describe a difficult situation, a kind of negative mood, and automatic thoughts. Users report the intensity of their negative mood on a scale from 0 (not stressed at all) to 100 (the most stressed they have ever felt).

- **Correcting Automatic Thoughts**: Through Socratic questioning, the agent helps the user examine their automatic thoughts by comparing them with factual evidence. This step aims to increase awareness of overlooked facts and encourage a more objective perspective.
- **Rethinking Balanced Alternative Thoughts**: Based on insights gained from correcting automatic thoughts, the user composes new, balanced thoughts. The agent then prompts the user to reassess their mood intensity, expecting a reduction in negative emotions.

4.2 Dialogue Scenario that Incorporates Socratic Questioning

To implement Socratic questioning, we used a pool of 21 flexible question templates that can be applied to various concerns and situations. These templates encourage users to reflect on their thought patterns by asking questions like:

- "Why do you think that way?"
- "What evidence supports or contradicts this thought?"
- "Have you considered other perspectives?"
- "How might someone else view this situation?"

The agent selects whether to add a question based on the estimated psychological distress, promoting deeper contemplation and cognitive restructuring.

4.3 Psychological Distress Detection Model

A critical component of the system is the psychological distress detection model, which estimates the user's level of distress in real-time during the CBT session. We adapted a deep learning architecture based on LSTM (Long Short-term Memory) to classify distress levels using transcription of user utterances.

Due to the scarcity of Japanese-language datasets for this task, we employed a combination of pre-training and transfer learning:

- **Pre-training**: We translated English datasets (DAIC-WOZ [15] and DailyDialog [16]) into Japanese using a Transformer-based translation model. The model was pre-trained on this translated data, maintaining equivalent performance levels despite the language change.
- **Transfer Learning**: We constructed a Japanese CBT dataset using crowd-sourcing, with responses labeled based on the K6 scale [14]. The model was fine-tuned using this dataset to detect distress levels accurately during CBT sessions.

The final model achieved an accuracy of 75%, with precision and recall scores indicating reliable performance. By incorporating this distress detection model, the agent can adjust the number of Socratic questions posed during the session:

- **If distress is detected**: The agent continues to ask an additional Socratic question to further aid cognitive restructuring.
- **If no distress is detected**: The agent proceeds to the next phase of the therapy session.

This real-time adaptation ensures that each session is personalized to the user's psychological state, enhancing engagement and therapeutic efficacy.

4.4 System Workflow

The interaction begins with the agent greeting the user and explaining the session's objectives. The user is guided to identify a troubling situation, report their mood and mood intensity, and express their automatic thoughts. Throughout the session, the agent understands user inputs, manages dialogue flow, and selects appropriate responses. The distress detection model analyzes user responses after each Socratic question to determine whether to continue with additional questions or move forward. This loop continues until the model indicates a reduction in distress or the maximum number of questions is reached. By adjusting the interaction based on real-time detections, the agent can provide a guide that aligns with the user's needs and readiness to rethink an alternative thought.

5 Experiment: Does Adapting Agent Responses to User Distress Improve CBT Effectiveness?

Figure 1 illustrates the experimental conditions. To evaluate the effectiveness of our adaptive CBT system, we conducted an experiment comparing two conditions: one where the number of Socratic questions was adapted based on the detected level of psychological distress (**adaptive condition**), and another where the number was randomly assigned (**random condition**).

5.1 Participants

The study involved 49 participants aged between 18 and 65, all of whom were native Japanese speakers with no hearing impairments. Participants were randomly assigned to either the adaptive condition (25 participants) or the random condition

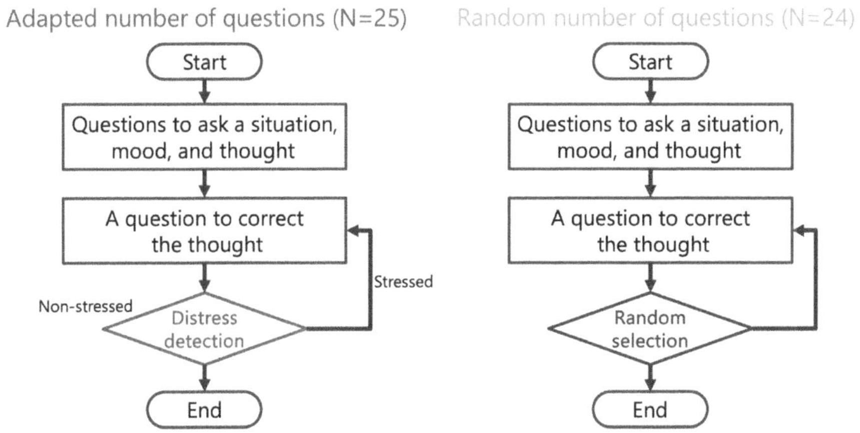

Fig. 1 Two experimental conditions. The adapted number of questions condition, which includes the psychological distress detection model, versus the random number of questions condition, which does not include the distress detection model

Table 1 Participants' demographics and baseline characteristics ($N = 49$)

Characteristics	Adapted number of questions condition	Random number of questions condition
Total number of participants, *n*	25	24
Sex		
Male, *n* (%)	12 (48)	13 (54)
Female, *n* (%)	13 (52)	11 (46)
Age (y), mean (SD)	41.72 (12.79)	38.88 (14.89)
K6[a], mean (SD)	4.08 (4.31)	4.38 (3.10)

[a] K6: Kessler psychological distress scale

(24 participants). One participant in the adaptive condition had a history of mental health issues but was in remission at the time of the study. Table 1 summarizes the participants' demographics and baseline characteristics.

Before the experiment, an experimenter explained this to the participants who signed the consent forms. They then completed the K6 questionnaire and read a publicly available leaflet explaining CBT [17]. The experiment was completed within 1 h, including its briefing and preparation.

5.2 *Measures*

We employed several measures to assess therapeutic outcomes:

- **Psychological Distress**: Measured using the K6 scale [14] before and after the session to assess the level of psychological distress. This scale consists of six self-report items. Each item is rated on a scale from 0 (none of the time) to 4 (all of the time), yielding a total score ranging from 0 to 24.
- **Cognitive Change**: Assessed using the Cognitive Change-Immediate scale [18], evaluating the extent of cognitive shifts experienced during the session. This scale consists of five self-report items. Each item is rated on a scale from 0 (not at all) to 6 (completely), yielding a total score ranging from 0 to 30.
- **Mood Change**: Participants reported their mood intensity on a scale from 0 to 100 before and after cognitive restructuring, indicating the severity of negative emotions.

5.3 Results

The adaptive condition showed significant improvements in psychological distress and mood compared to the random condition.

Psychological Distress: Participants in the adaptive condition experienced a greater reduction in K6 scores post-session (mean change = 1.04) compared to the random condition (mean change = 0.08). The post-session distress levels were significantly lower in the adaptive condition (Cliff's delta = −0.17, $p = 0.04$; one-sided Mann-Whitney U test). See Fig. 2.

Mood Change: A larger decrease in negative mood intensity was observed in the adaptive condition, with significant reductions after the session (Cliff's delta = −0.08, $p = 0.16$; one-sided Mann-Whitney U test).

Cognitive Change: While both conditions showed improvements, the adaptive condition demonstrated a trend toward greater cognitive change, though not statistically significant (Cliff's delta = 0.12, $p = 0.07$; one-sided Mann-Whitney U test). See Fig. 2.

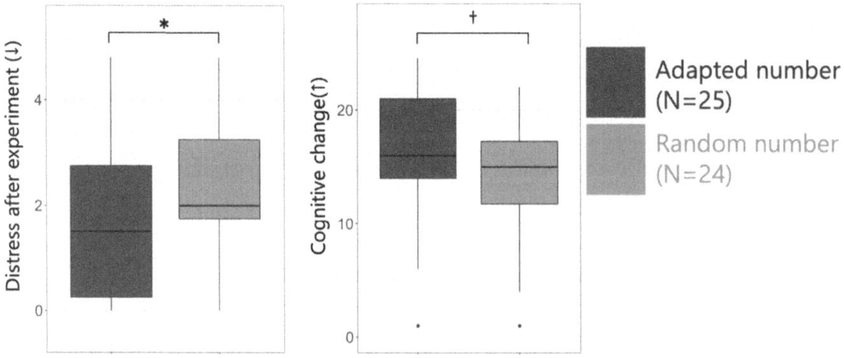

Fig. 2 Pre- and post-session measures for the adapted and random number of questions conditions

These results suggest that ECAs adapting their questioning strategies based on real-time distress detection achieve superior outcomes in reducing psychological distress compared to the random number conditon.

Additionally, we evaluated the performance of the distress detection model. In the adaptive condition, the model correctly identified non-distressed states in 72% of instances. Participants whose distress levels were accurately detected showed greater cognitive change compared to the random condition, revealing the importance of accurate distress detection.

6 Discussion and Implications for Future CBT Systems

The findings imply the importance of adapting response selection in CBT with an ECA. Adapting the number and type of Socratic questions based on users' psychological states enhances the efficacy of the cognitive restructuring, leading to greater reductions in distress and negative moods.

6.1 Importance of Accurate Distress Detection

The effectiveness of the adaptive system hinges on the accuracy of the psychological distress detection model. Our results indicate that correctly identifying the user's distress level is crucial for optimizing the number of questions and, consequently, the therapeutic outcome. Participants whose distress levels were accurately detected experienced more significant cognitive changes, suggesting that precise real-time detections enable the agent to adapt interventions effectively.

Future systems should focus on improving detection models, possibly by incorporating multimodal data such as speech, facial expressions, and physiological signals. Enhancing the model's accuracy can lead to more personalized and effective therapeutic interactions.

6.2 Understanding Interaction from Multifaceted Perspectives

While the adaptive system improved distress levels, its impact on cognitive change was less pronounced. This indicates a need for more nuanced adaptations that consider not only emotional states but also cognitive processes. Future research should explore methods to enhance both cognitive and emotional outcomes, possibly by adapting the content and complexity of questions.

Integrating user feedback mechanisms and adjusting the questioning strategy based on cognitive indicators can further personalize the interaction. For example, assessing the user's engagement level or comprehension may help the agent determine when to provide additional support or move forward.

7 Conclusion

The integration of the adaptive questioning method in ECAs represents a significant advancement in the delivery of CBT. By adapting questions based on real-time psychological distress detection, ECAs can provide more personalized and effective therapy sessions. This approach not only improves therapeutic outcomes but also enhances user engagement and satisfaction.

This study demonstrates that adapting to a user's psychological state by modulating the number of Socratic questions can significantly reduce psychological distress compared to non-adaptive methods. These findings align with clinical insights emphasizing the importance of personalized interventions in mental health care.

Acknowledgements Finding was provided by ANR-JST-CREST TAPAS [grant number ANR-19-JSTS-0001] project.

This chapter is an extension of the PhD thesis of the first author which was done at Nara Institute of Science and Technology

References

1. Beck AT. Cognitive therapy of depression. Guilford Press, (1979)
2. J.S. Beck, Cognitive behavior therapy, third edition: basics and beyond. Guilford Publications, (2020)
3. D. Greenberger, C.A. Padesky, Mind over mood, second edition: change how you feel by changing the way you think. Guilford Publications, (2015)
4. M. Freeman, The world mental health report: transforming mental health for all. World Psychiatry **21**, 391–392 (2022)
5. K. Denecke, N. Schmid, S. Nüssli, Implementation of cognitive behavioral therapy in e-mental health apps: literature review. J. Med. Internet Res. **24**, e27791 (2022)
6. L. Laranjo, A.G. Dunn, H.L. Tong, A.B. Kocaballi, J. Chen, R. Bashir et al., Conversational agents in healthcare: a systematic review. J. Am. Med. Inform. Assoc. **25**, 1248–1258 (2018)
7. A.A. Abd-Alrazaq, A. Rababeh, M. Alajlani, B.M. Bewick, M. Househ, Effectiveness and safety of using chatbots to improve mental health: systematic review and meta-analysis. J. Med. Internet Res. **22**, e16021 (2020)
8. B. Lugrin, C. Pelachaud, D. Traum, *The handbook on socially interactive agents: 20 years of research on embodied conversational agents, intelligent virtual agents, and social robotics: Methods, behavior, cognition.* New York, NY: Association of Computing Machinery, (2021) vol. 1

9. G.I. Clark, S.J. Egan, The socratic method in cognitive behavioural therapy: a narrative review. Cognit Ther Res. **39**, 863–879 (2015)
10. E. Kimani, T. Bickmore, H. Trinh, P. Pedrelli, *You'll be Great: Virtual Agent-based Cognitive Restructuring to Reduce Public Speaking Anxiety*. 2019 8th International Conference on Affective Computing and Intelligent Interaction (ACII). (2019), pp. 641–647
11. K. Shidara, H. Tanaka, H. Adachi, D. Kanayama, Y. Sakagami, T. Kudo et al., Automatic thoughts and facial expressions in cognitive restructuring with virtual agents. Front. Comput. Sci. (2022). https://doi.org/10.3389/fcomp.2022.762424
12. K. Shidara, H. Tanaka, H. Adachi, D. Kanayama, T. Kudo, S. Nakamura, Adapting the number of questions based on detected psychological distress for cognitive behavioral therapy with an embodied conversational agent: Comparative study. JMIR Form. Res. **8**, e50056 (2024)
13. C. Li, C. Braud, M. Amblard, Multi-task learning for depression detection in dialogs. (2022), pp. 68–75
14. T.A. Furukawa, R.C. Kessler, T. Slade, G. Andrews, The performance of the K6 and K10 screening scales for psychological distress in the Australian National Survey of Mental Health and Well-Being. Psychol. Med. **33**, 357–362 (2003)
15. J. Gratch, R. Artstein, G. Lucas, G. Stratou, S. Scherer, A. Nazarian, et al. The distress analysis interview corpus of human and computer interviews. (2014), pp. 3123–3128
16. Y. Li, H. Su, X. Shen, W. Li, Z. Cao, S. Niu, *DailyDialog: A Manually Labelled Multi-turn Dialogue Dataset. Proceedings of the Eighth International Joint Conference on Natural Language Processing (Volume 1: Long Papers)*. Taipei, Taiwan: Asian Federation of Natural Language Processing, (2017), pp. 986–995
17. Y. Ono, In: Leaflet: using cognitive behavior therapy to improve mental skills. [Internet]. [Cited 3 Jun 2023]. Available: https://www.cbtjp.net/downloads/skillup/
18. I.D. Schmidt, B.J. Pfeifer, D.R. Strunk, Putting the "cognitive" back in cognitive therapy: Sustained cognitive change as a mediator of in-session insights and depressive symptom improvement. J. Consult. Clin. Psychol. **87**, 446–456 (2019)

Introduces Evaluation

Validation of Developed Automated SST System

Masato Honda, Kosuke Okazaki, and Hiroki Tanaka

Abstract This study aims to validate an automated social skills training (SST) system designed to assist individuals with distinct social communication challenges. Specifically, it targets those diagnosed with schizophrenia, who often struggle with social withdrawal, flat affect, and difficulty in interpreting social cues, as well as individuals with autism spectrum disorder, who typically face challenges in understanding nonverbal communication, maintaining reciprocal conversations, and adapting to social norms. The system is intended to help these individuals objectively assess their social interactions, learn appropriate social cues, and develop strategies to improve their communication skills in various social contexts. We conducted two key verifications: (1) comparing the improvement in social skills between a group of healthy adults trained with our SST system and a wait-list control group of healthy adults who received no intervention during the study period and (2) assessing the effectiveness of our SST system compared to traditional human–human SST. This chapter presents an analysis of the first verification, which has been completed, and outlines the experimental design for the second, which is currently in progress. Our findings demonstrate the effectiveness of the automated SST system over a four-week training period, with significant improvements in general self-efficacy, reduction in state anxiety, and enhanced speech clarity in the trained group.

M. Honda (✉) · K. Okazaki
Department of Psychiatry, Nara Medical University, Kashihara, Japan
e-mail: masato.h@naramed-u.ac.jp

K. Okazaki
e-mail: okazaki-k@heartland.or.jp

K. Okazaki
Children's Mental Health Center, Shigisan Hospital, Nara, Japan

H. Tanaka
Division of Arts and Sciences, International Christian University, Mitaka, Japan
e-mail: hiroki.tanaka@icu.ac.jp

S. Nakamura (ed.), *Multimodal Interaction Technologies for Training Affective Social Skills*, https://doi.org/10.1007/978-981-96-1313-7_12

1 Introduction

Social skills training (SST) is a well-established method for teaching appropriate social and communication skills, strengthening social self-efficacy, and reducing social anxiety [1, 2]. Traditionally conducted by human trainers, SST follows structured approaches, such as the model proposed by Bellack et al. [3], which incorporates the core principles of social learning theory: modeling, shaping, reinforcement, overlearning, and generalization.

However, human-led SST faces limitations in cost-effectiveness and accessibility, particularly in areas where professional trainers are scarce. To address these challenges, researchers have been exploring automated SST using conversational agents or robots, aiming to provide SST anytime and anywhere [4–6]. These efforts have led to the development of automated SST systems [7–12] that simulate human-led SST [13–15].

Our study developed an automated SST system adhering to Bellack et al. training model, incorporating a conversational agent capable of speech recognition, response selection, speech synthesis, and generation of nonverbal behaviors. This system builds upon previous research in automated SST, including video modeling of human behavior, automatic real-time behavior recognition, and feedback [13, 15].

The potential of automated SST systems has been evaluated in terms of training effect by short-term single-group intervention [13], acceptability [14], and social self-efficacy [15]. However, there has been no thorough evaluation of the long-term effects of such SST systems or a comparison with a control group. This study aims to address this gap by validating our SST system for members of the general population over a four-week period.

2 Methods

2.1 Study Design

We employed a nonrandomized comparative design with two groups:

1. System-trained group (Group 1)
2. Non-trained control group (Group 2)

Initially, 26 healthy Japanese participants aged 20–35 years were recruited, with 13 participants in each group and a balanced gender ratio. The participants were not informed of the tasks of the other group. The trainers and third-party raters did not know to which group a participant belonged.

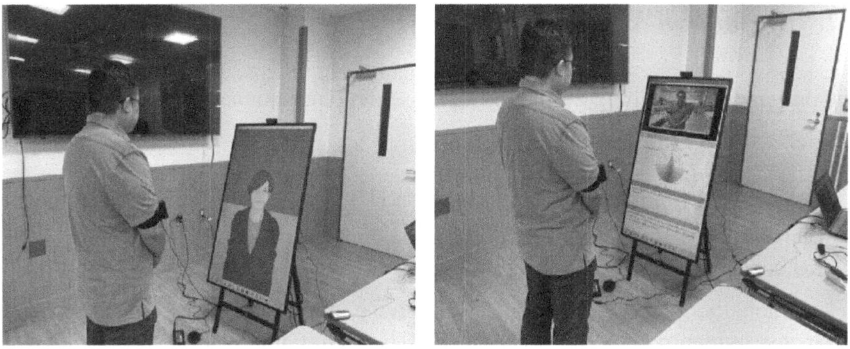

Fig. 1 Social skills training system (left: role-playing; right: feedback) [34]

2.2 Automated SST System

The automated SST system utilized the Greta platform [4] with a conversational agent named Rei, incorporating speech recognition, response selection, speech synthesis, and nonverbal behavior generation. Four basic SST tasks were created based on Bellack's method:

1. Declining requests
2. Listening to others
3. Making requests
4. Expressing positive feelings

The system includes video modeling of human behavior, automatic real-time behavior recognition, and a feedback function. We constructed a score evaluator from role-play videos and automatically predicted seven items: eye contact, body orientation, facial expression, vocal variation, clarity, fluency, and social appropriateness. These were rated by psychiatrist evaluators on a 5-point scale.

As shown in Fig. 1, the system provides a realistic role-playing environment with a virtual agent (left) and offers detailed feedback through a radar chart and textual comments (right). This visual feedback helps participants understand their performance level and areas needing improvement.

2.3 Training Protocol

Group 1 participants visited the experiment space at Nara Institute of Science and Technology weekly for four weeks. Each 30-min training session covered three of the four basic skills. The system operated automatically, but an examiner was present to ensure proper functioning.

2.4 Evaluation Measures

The pre- and post-training evaluations used several questionnaires:

1. General self-efficacy scale [16, 17]
2. Social responsiveness scale-2 [18, 19]
3. State-trait anxiety inventory (STAI) [20, 21]
4. Liebowitz social anxiety scale [22, 23]
5. Kikuchi scale of social skills-18 [24]

Additionally, a performance test involving three role-play scenarios was conducted, video-recorded, and evaluated by blind third-party trainers. These scenarios required social cognition and expression of the participants in new role-play situations: (1) understanding and expressing empathic behaviors, (2) self-disclosure, and (3) social problem-solving with one's mother.

2.5 Statistical Analysis

Statistical analysis employed nonparametric Wilcoxon Rank Sum tests to compare pre- and post-training evaluations. Effect sizes were calculated, and intraclass correlation coefficients assessed agreement between third-party raters.

3 Results

Of the 26 recruited participants, 18 completed the experiment (9 in each group). Key findings from the study, as reported in Tanaka et al. [34], include:

General Self-Efficacy: Group 1 (system-trained) showed significant improvement compared to Group 2 ($P = 0.02$, effect size $r = 0.53$).

State Anxiety: Group 1 demonstrated a significant decrease in state anxiety presence compared to Group 2 ($P = 0.04$, $r = 0.49$), as measured by the State-Trait Anxiety Inventory (STAI).

Speech Clarity: Third-party ratings revealed significant improvement for Group 1 compared to Group 2 ($P = 0.03$, $r = 0.30$).

Other measures showed trends toward improvement in Group 1, including decreased anxiety during role-play performance, improved planning skills, and enhanced body direction and distance in role-play scenarios, although these did not reach statistical significance.

The intraclass correlation coefficients between third-party raters showed good agreement across all evaluated aspects (ranging from 0.78 to 0.89, all $P < 0.001$).

Table 1, adapted from Tanaka et al. [34], presents a comprehensive overview of the evaluation outcomes, comparing the pre-training evaluation and the difference between post- and pre-training evaluations for both groups. The table includes results from the questionnaires used, that is, the General Self-Efficacy Scale, STAI, Liebowitz Social Anxiety Scale (LSAS), Social Responsiveness Scale-2 (SRS-2), and Kikuchi Scale of Social Skills-18 (KiSS-18), as well as the results of performance tests evaluated by third-party raters.

These results suggest that the automated SST system had a positive impact on participants' social skills, particularly in terms of general self-efficacy, state anxiety, and speech clarity. The significant improvements observed in the system-trained group (Group 1) compared to the non-trained group (Group 2) provide initial evidence for the effectiveness of the automated SST system.

4 Discussion

Our findings demonstrate the effectiveness of the proposed automated SST system over a four-week training period. Significant improvements in general self-efficacy, a reduction in state anxiety, and enhanced speech clarity in the trained group align with traditional SST goals.

The improvement in self-efficacy is particularly noteworthy, since it is fundamental to behavioral change according to Bandura's theory [25]. The system's positive reinforcement likely contributed to this outcome. The reduction in state anxiety may be attributed to the safe and successful experiences provided by role-playing with the conversational agent.

Our SST system praises the learner and provides positive reinforcement, affecting gains in self-efficacy [15, 26]. Moreover, it can be argued that our SST strengthens self-efficacy, leading to behavioral modification [25]. We found reductions in both state anxiety and anxiety over role-playing, which we attribute to the safety of role-playing with the conversational agent as well as the successful user experiences the system provides. Another study also found that if encouragement and successful experiences are present, the user feels an increased sense of trust, security, and safety and reduced tension, threat, and anxiety [27].

Our primary outcome was improved speech clarity. Our SST system includes feedback with concrete suggestions for behavior, which likely leads to improvement in speech clarity. Previous work also reported an improved frequency of positive social behavior through human–human SST [28]. Heinssen et al. [29] reported that participants learned, retained, and generalized new social skills through human SST.

4.1 Limitations

While our results are promising, several limitations should be noted:

1. The small sample size and focus on a healthy population limit generalizability.
2. The nonrandomized design may have introduced selection bias.

Table 1 Nonparametric analysis of rank sum test for differences between groups. Effect size *r* and *P* values correspond to post–pre values between the two groups.*

	Pretraining		Posttraining		Posttraining-pretraining difference		Effect size *r*	*P* Value
	Group 1 (*n* = 9), mean (SD)	Group 2 (*n* = 9), mean (SD)	Group 1 (*n* = 9), mean (SD)	Group 2 (*n* = 9), mean (SD)	Group 1 (*n* = 9), mean (SD)	Group 2 (*n* = 9), mean (SD)		
General self-efficacy scale								
Total	8.22 (3.96)	7.44 (4.77)	8.67 (3.61)	6.22 (4.55)	0.44 (3.97)	– 1.22 (1.09)	0.42	0.07[a]
Normalized score	2.44 (1.13)	2.67 (1.22)	2.89 (1.05)	2.22 (1.30)	0.44 (1.13)	– 0.44 (0.53)	0.53	0.02[b]
STAI[c] (inverse[d])								
Total (state)	42.00 (7.97)	41.89 (10.36)	39.67 (9.19)	43.89 (9.62)	– 2.33 (5.17)	2.00 (6.89)	0.36	0.12
State anxiety presence	44.44 (5.79)	43.00 (5.59)	42.56 (8.35)	45.22 (7.07)	– 1.89 (4.48)	2.22 (6.26)	0.49	0.04[b]
State anxiety absence	44.44 (7.94)	46.22 (12.40)	42.67 (6.93)	46.89 (9.25)	– 1.78 (5.67)	0.67 (6.78)	0.16	0.50
Total (trait)	47.33 (10.51)	49.00 (12.54)	46.56 (9.98)	49.78 (11.38)	– 0.78 (9.71)	0.78 (5.38)	0.12	0.62
Trait anxiety presence	51.67 (11.19)	52.00 (11.28)	49.78 (9.36)	51.78 (10.23)	– 1.89 (10.68)	– 0.22 (5.04)	0.13	0.59
Trait anxiety absence	40.67 (8.58)	43.89 (11.56)	41.78 (8.47)	45.89 (10.06)	1.11 (7.10)	2.00 (4.80)	0.16	0.50
LSAS[e] (inversed)								
Total	49.78 (26.47)	46.22 (30.76)	56.00 (31.14)	51.11 (33.14)	6.22 (29.28)	4.89 (9.99)	0.15	0.52
Total (anxiety)	24.00 (13.02)	27.00 (14.73)	27.44 (14.73)	29.33 (18.81)	3.44 (17.05)	2.33 (6.48)	0.09	0.71
Performance anxiety	11.67 (6.52)	11.67 (9.77)	13.89 (7.01)	13.56 (10.19)	2.22 (8.64)	1.89 (2.42)	0.19	0.43
Social anxiety[f]	12.33 (6.76)	15.33 (9.29)	13.56 (8.23)	15.78 (9.32)	1.22 (8.66)	0.44 (5.36)	0.05	0.82
Total (avoidance)	25.78 (16.02)	19.22 (13.75)	28.33 (17.30)	21.78 (15.59)	2.56 (13.25)	2.56 (6.02)	0.13	0.58
Performance avoidance	11.78 (8.26)	8.44 (7.13)	13.44 (7.63)	9.78 (7.81)	1.67 (6.36)	1.33 (3.54)	0.15	0.53
Social avoidance	14.00 (7.98)	10.78 (7.07)	14.89 (9.84)	12.00 (8.03)	0.89 (7.59)	1.22 (2.86)	0.14	0.55
SRS-2[g] (inversed)								
Total	69.78 (22.73)	67.89 (36.14)	70.78 (24.55)	67.67 (34.06)	1.00 (15.38)	– 0.22 (7.93)	0.11	0.65

(continued)

Table 1 (continued)

	Pretraining		Posttraining		Posttraining-pretraining difference		Effect size *r*	*P* Value
	Group 1 (*n* = 9), mean (SD)	Group 2 (*n* = 9), mean (SD)	Group 1 (*n* = 9), mean (SD)	Group 2 (*n* = 9), mean (SD)	Group 1 (*n* = 9), mean (SD)	Group 2 (*n* = 9), mean (SD)		
Awareness	8.56 (3.43)	7.67 (4.21)	9.00 (2.92)	7.56 (3.75)	0.44 (0.51)	− 0.11 (1.83)	0.06	0.80
Cognition	12.89 (4.94)	14.22 (6.14)	11.89 (5.13)	13.22 (6.04)	− 1.00 (4.33)	− 1.00 (2.18)	0.10	0.67
Communication	21.67 (9.49)	21.33 (14.06)	21.33 (8.62)	20.22 (12.25)	− 0.33 (6.06)	− 1.11 (3.92)	0.08	0.73
Motivation	12.22 (3.56)	13.56 (7.09)	14.67 (4.87)	15.89 (7.46)	2.44 (5.83)	2.33 (3.24)	0.28	0.22
Repetitive and restricted behaviours	14.44 (7.40)	11.11 (7.06)	13.89 (7.24)	10.78 (6.20)	− 0.56 (4.13)	− 0.33 (3.12)	0.11	0.64
KiSS-18 [h]								
Total	59.89 (12.33)	60.00 (16.40)	61.44 (11.50)	61.22 (12.84)	1.56 (6.65)	1.22 (5.70)	0.17	0.48
Basic skills	9.22 (3.27)	9.44 (2.79)	9.89 (3.22)	10.22 (2.82)	0.67 (1.12)	0.78 (0.83)	0.11	0.65
Advanced skills	10.56 (2.40)	10.67 (2.69)	10.78 (2.49)	11.11 (2.80)	0.22 (2.39)	0.44 (1.01)	0.09	0.71
Emotion processing	9.33 (2.83)	9.56 (4.03)	9.67 (2.60)	9.44 (1.88)	0.33 (1.80)	− 0.11 (2.26)	0.26	0.27
Offensive	9.22 (2.33)	8.56 (3.28)	9.67 (2.24)	9.33 (2.40)	0.44 (1.67)	0.78 (1.92)	0.10	0.66
Stress coping	10.11 (2.71)	10.11 (3.37)	9.78 (2.68)	10.00 (3.20)	− 0.33 (1.73)	− 0.11 (2.09)	0.15	0.52
Planning	11.44 (1.81)	11.67 (1.09)	11.67 (1.87)	11.11 (2.26)	0.22 (1.09)	− 0.56 (1.33)	0.41	0.08[a]
Performance test [i]								
Anxiety (inversed)	2.22 (0.97)	2.25 (0.98)	1.93 (0.73)	2.26 (0.76)	− 0.30 (0.99)	0 (0.73)	0.23	0.08[a]
Self-efficacy[f]	2.56 (1.09)	2.44 (0.93)	2.33 (0.88)	2.44 (0.85)	− 0.22 (0.75)	0 (0.78)	0.03	0.84
Eye contact	4.35 (1.08)	4.52 (0.69)	4.37 (1.09)	4.48 (0.75)	0.02 (0.35)	− 0.04 (0.40)	0.17	0.21
Body direction and distance	4.44 (0.92)	4.61 (0.64)	4.52 (0.80)	4.56 (0.67)	0.07 (0.38)	− 0.06 (0.35)	0.22	0.10

(continued)

Table 1 (continued)

	Pretraining		Posttraining		Posttraining-pretraining difference		Effect size r	P Value
	Group 1 (n = 9), mean (SD)	Group 2 (n = 9), mean (SD)	Group 1 (n = 9), mean (SD)	Group 2 (n = 9), mean (SD)	Group 1 (n = 9), mean (SD)	Group 2 (n = 9), mean (SD)		
Facial expression	3.96 (1.10)	4.02 (0.90)	4.04 (0.96)	4.07 (0.89)	0.07 (0.58)	0.06 (0.42)	0.10	0.46
Vocal variation	4.26 (1.10)	4.48 (0.67)	4.37 (0.93)	4.57 (0.74)	0.11 (0.47)	0.09 (0.37)	0.07	0.61
Clarity	4.17 (1.02)	4.46 (0.72)	4.48 (0.86)	4.46 (0.82)	0.31 (0.57)	0 (0.54)	0.30	0.03[b]
Fluency	4.11 (1.11)	4.39 (0.68)	4.37 (0.96)	4.54 (0.76)	0.26 (0.67)	0.15 (0.48)	0.14	0.30
Social appropriateness	4.11 (1.11)	4.39 (0.68)	4.37 (0.96)	4.54 (0.76)	0.26 (0.67)	0.15 (0.48)	0.14	0.29

[a] $P < 0.10$
[b] $P < 0.05$
[c] STAI: State-trait anxiety inventory
[d] Inversed indicates that greater values show lesser skill and higher anxiety
[e] LSAS: Liebowitz social anxiety scale
[f] Note that self-efficacy and social anxiety were obtained from three role-plays
[g] SRS-2: Social Responsiveness scale–2
[h] KiSS-18: Kikuchi scale of social skills–18
[i] The performance test was conducted in a concatenation of three role-play scenarios
* Adapted from Tanaka et al. [34]

3. The short-term nature of the study does not address long-term skill retention or generalization.
4. The presence of an examiner during training sessions may have influenced participant behavior.
5. The study did not evaluate performance in emotion recognition tasks [30].
6. Some participants' scores did not change between the beginning and end of the training, which might be related to the boredom of repetitive training.

4.2 Future Directions

Future research directions should include:

1. Larger-scale studies with diverse populations, including individuals with autism spectrum disorder and schizophrenia.
2. Randomized controlled trials with longer follow-up periods.
3. Comparison of the automated SST system with traditional human–human SST.

4. Further refinement of the system, including more sophisticated behavior modeling and enhancement of the agent's naturalistic nonverbal behaviors.
5. Clarification of the optimal training duration and number of role-play repetitions.
6. Extension of the study to include children [31].
7. Development of a web-based SST system that could be used as a supplement to human SST.

5 Ongoing Research: Comparison with Human-Led SST

5.1 Experimental Design

We are currently conducting a study to compare the effectiveness of our automated SST system with traditional human-led SST. The study design includes:

- Subjects: Healthy individuals recruited from Nara Institute of Science and Technology students and through a staffing agency.
- Exclusion criteria: History of psychiatric outpatient treatment, epilepsy, neurological diseases, substance abuse, addiction, head trauma, and various eye conditions.
- Groups: 45 participants non-blindly randomized into three groups ($N = 15$ each):
- Waiting-list control group
- Human-led SST group
- System-led SST group

5.2 Training Protocol

- Duration: One month, with weekly one-hour sessions.
- Tasks: Four basic tasks (expressing feelings, refusing, making requests, and listening).

5.3 Evaluation Measures

Evaluations are conducted one week before and after training, including:

1. Role-plays with SST trainers, assessed using three items from the revised role-play evaluation scale.
2. Self-efficacy evaluation using the Japanese version of the General Self-Efficacy Scale [17].
3. Anxiety assessment using Japanese versions of the State-Trait Anxiety Inventory [21] and Liebowitz Social Anxiety Scale [23].

4. Social functioning evaluation using Kikuchi's Scale of Social Skills [24].
5. Pre-training assessment of social functional outcomes using the Specific Levels of Functioning Scale [32].
6. Pre-training evaluation of social cognition using the Emotion Discrimination Task [33].
7. SST trainers are experienced professionals with over three years of SST experience. Role-play evaluations are conducted blindly by trainers different from those who conducted the sessions.

Data analysis for this verification is currently in progress.

6 Conclusion

This research provides initial evidence for the efficacy of an automated SST system in improving social skills, enhancing self-efficacy, and reducing anxiety. These findings pave the way for more accessible and cost-effective SST interventions, potentially benefiting a wider range of individuals who require social skills development. Ongoing comparisons with human–human SST will further elucidate the potential of this automated system in clinical applications.

Our automated SST system offers a comprehensive approach to social skills training, combining realistic role-playing scenarios with detailed performance feedback. The results demonstrate the system's potential to improve various aspects of social functioning, particularly in areas such as self-efficacy, anxiety reduction, and speech clarity.

Future research will focus on refining the system, expanding its application to diverse populations, and comparing its effectiveness with traditional human-led SST. These efforts are expected to establish automated SST as a viable and accessible option for individuals seeking to improve their social skills, potentially revolutionizing the field of social skills training and therapy.

References

1. R.P. Liberman, K.T. Mueser, C.J. Wallace, Social skills training for schizophrenic individuals at risk for relapse. Am. J. Psychiatry **143**(4), 523–526 (1986)
2. K.O. Moe, A.M. Zeiss, Measuring self-efficacy expectations for social skills: a methodological inquiry. Cogn. Ther. Res. **6**(2), 191–205 (1982)
3. A.S. Bellack, K.T. Meuser, S. Gingerich, J. Agresta, *Social Skills Training for Schizophrenia: A Step-by-Step Guide* (Guilford Press, New York, NY, 1997), pp.637–638
4. C. Poggi, C. Pelachaud, F. de Rosis, V. Carofiglio, B. de Carolis Greta, A believable embodied conversational agent. In: Stock O, Zancanaro M, editors. Multimodal Intelligent Information Presentation. Dordrecht, (The Netherlands: Springer; 2005) pp. 3–5
5. D. Novick, I. Gris, Building rapport between human and ECA: a pilot study. 2014 Presented at: HCI 2014: International Conference on Human-Computer Interaction; June 22–27, (Heraklion, Crete, Greece 2014) p. 472–480

6. H. Kumazaki, Z. Warren, T. Muramatsu, Y. Yoshikawa, Y. Matsumoto, M. Miyao et al., A pilot study for robot appearance preferences among high-functioning individuals with autism spectrum disorder: implications for therapeutic use. PLoS ONE **12**(10), e0186581 (2017)
7. E.E. Soares, K. Bausback, C.L. Beard, M. Higinbotham, E.L. Bunge, G.W. Gengoux, Social skills training for autism spectrum disorder: a meta-analysis of in-person and technological interventions. J. Technol. Behav. Sci. **6**(1), 166–180 (2021)
8. M.R. Ali, Z. Razavi, A.A. Mamum, R. Langevin, B. Kane, R. Rawassizadeh, et al. A virtual conversational agent for teens with autism: experimental results and design lessons. arXiv. Preprint posted online on November 7, (2018)
9. M. Hoque, M. Courgeon, J.C. Martin, B. Multin, R.W. Picard, MACH: my automated conversation coach. 2013 Sep 8 Presented at: ACM International Joint Conference on Pervasive and Ubiquitous Computing (UbiComp '13); September 8–12, (Zurich, Switzerland, 2013) p. 697–706
10. M. Esposito, J. Sloan, A. Tancredi, G. Gerardi, P. Postiglione, F. Fotia et al., Using tablet applications for children with autism to increase their cognitive and social skills. J. Spec. Educ. Technol. **32**(4), 199–209 (2017)
11. M.R. Ali, E. Hoque, Social skills training with virtual assistant and real-time feedback. 2017 Sep 11 Presented at: UbiComp '17: the 2017 ACM International Joint Conference on Pervasive and Ubiquitous Computing; September 11–15, (Maui, Hawaii, 2017) p. 325–329.
12. S. Parsons, P. Mitchell, The potential of virtual reality in social skills training for people with autistic spectrum disorders. J. Intellect. Disabil. Res. **46**(Pt 5), 430–443 (2002)
13. H. Tanaka, H. Negoro, H. Iwasaka, S. Nakamura, Embodied conversational agents for multimo
14. H. Tanaka, H. Negoro, H. Iwasaka, S. Nakamura, Embodied conversational agents for multimodal automated social skills training in people with autism spectrum disorders. PLoS ONE **12**(8), e0182151 (2017)
15. H. Tanaka, S. Nakamura, The acceptability of virtual characters as social skills trainers: usability study. JMIR Hum. Factors **9**(1), e35358 (2022)
16. H. Tanaka, H. Iwasaka, Y. Matsuda, K. Okazaki, S. Nakamura, Analyzing self-efficacy and summary feedback in automated social skills training. IEEE Open J. Eng. Med. Biol. **27**(2), 65–70 (2021)
17. A. Luszczynska, U. Scholz, R. Schwarzer, The general self-efficacy scale: multicultural validation studies. J. Psychol. **139**(5), 439–457 (2005)
18. Y. Sakano, T. Mitsuhiko, The general self-efficacy scale (GSES): scale development and validation article in Japanese. Jpn. J. Behav. Therapy **12**(1), 73–82 (1986)
19. J.N. Constantino, C.P.Gruber, Social responsiveness scale: SRS-2. Torrance, CA: Western Psychological Services, (2012)
20. Y. Kamio, N. Inada, A. Moriwaki, M. Kuroda, T. Koyama, H. Tsujii et al., Quantitative autistic traits ascertained in a national survey of 22 529 Japanese schoolchildren. Acta Psychiatr. Scand. **128**(1), 45–53 (2013)
21. C.D. Spielberger, State-Trait Anxiety Inventory for Adults. APA PsycTests, (1983)
22. N. Hidano, M. Fukuhara, M. Iwawaki, S. Soga, C.D. Spielberger, State Trait Anxiety Inventory (Form JYZ). Article in Japanese. Tokyo, Japan: Japan UNI Agency, (2000)
23. M.R. Liebowitz, Social phobia. Mod. Probl. Pharmacopsychiatry **22**, 141–173 (1987)
24. S. Asakura, S. Inoue, F. Sasaki, Y. Sasaki, N. Kitagawa, T. Inoue et al., Reliability and validity of the Japanese version of the Liebowitz social anxiety scale. Seishin Igaku **44**(10), 1077–1084 (2002)
25. K. Kikuchi, The social skills are measured. Article in Japanese. In: Shakaiteki-sukiru-wo-hakaru-kiss-18 handbook. The handbook of KiSS-18. Tokyo, Japan: Kawashima, (2007)
26. A. Bandura, Self-efficacy: toward a unifying theory of behavioral change. Psychol. Rev. **84**(2), 191–215 (1977)
27. D.H. Schunk, Self-efficacy and cognitive achievement: implications for students with learning problems. J. Learn. Disabil. **22**(1), 14–22 (1989)
28. M.J. Lambert, A.E. Bergin, S.L. Garfield, The effectiveness of psychotherapy. In: Encyclopedia of Psychotherapy, Vol. 1. (Cambridge, MA: Academic Press 1994) pp. 709–714

29. N.K. Yang, J.L. Schaller, T. Huang, M.H. Wang, S. Tsai, Enhancing appropriate social behaviors for children with autism in general education classrooms: an analysis of six cases. Educ. Train. Dev. Disabil. **38**(4), 405–416 (2003)
30. R.K. Heinssen, R.P. Liberman, A. Kopelowicz, Psychosocial skills training for schizophrenia: lessons from the laboratory. Schizophr. Bull. **26**(1), 21–46 (2000)
31. P. Ekman, W.V. Friesen, *Pictures of Facial Affect* (Consulting Psychologists Press, Palo Alto, CA, 1976)
32. K. Yamamuro, T. Ota, J. Iida, Y. Nakanishi, Y. Suehiro, H. Matsuura et al., Event-related potentials correlate with the severity of child and adolescent patients with attention deficit/ hyperactivity disorder. Neuropsychobiology **73**(3), 131–138 (2016)
33. L.C. Schneider, E.L. Struening, SLOF: a behavioral rating scale for assessing the mentally ill. Soc. Work Res. Abs. **19**(3), 9–21 (1983)
34. S. Baron-Cohen, S. Wheelwright, J. Hill, Y. Raste, I. Plumb, The, reading the mind in the eyes test revised version: a study with normal adults, and adults with Asperger syndrome or high-functioning autism. J. Child Psychol. Psychiatry **42**(2), 241–251 (2001)